Aspen's Orthopaedic Physical Therapy Series

# SHOULDER
## PATHOPHYSIOLOGY
### Rehabilitation and Treatment

## Scott V. Haig, MD

Assistant Clinical Professor of Orthopaedics
College of Physicians and Surgeons
Columbia University
New York, New York

Assistant Attending
Orthopaedic Surgery
Columbia Presbyterian Medical Center
New York, New York

Director
Adult Orthopaedics
Helen Hayes Hospital
Haverstraw, New York

Attending Orthopaedic Surgeon
Lawrence Hospital
Bronxville, New York

AN ASPEN PUBLICATION®
Aspen Publishers, Inc.
Gaithersburg, Maryland
1996

Library of Congress Cataloging-in-Publication Data
Haig, Scott Vanderwink.
Shoulder pathophysiology : rehabilitation and treatment/
Scott V. Haig.
p.  cm. — (Aspen's orthopaedic physical therapy series)
Includes bibliographical references and index.
ISBN 0-8342-0622-6
1. Shoulder—Pathophysiology.
2. Shoulder joint—Pathophysiology.
3. Shoulder—Wounds and injuries.
4. Shoulder joint—Wounds and injuries.
5. Shoulder joint—Diseases.
6. Shoulder—Diseases.
I. Title. II. Series.
[DNLM: 1. Shoulder Joint—physiopathology.
2. Shoulder—physiopathology. 3. Joint Diseases.
4. Arm Injuries. 5. Athletic Injuries. WE 810 H149s 1996]
RD557.5.H35      1996
617.5'72—dc20
DNLM/DLC
for Library of Congress
95-14128
CIP

Aspen Publishers, Inc., grants permission for photocopying for limited personal or internal use. This consent does not extend to other kinds of copying, such as copying for general distribution, for advertising or promotional purposes, for creating new collective works, or for resale. For information, address Aspen Publishers, Inc., Permissions Department, 200 Orchard Ridge Drive, Suite 200, Gaithersburg, Maryland 20878.

The authors have made every effort to ensure the accuracy of the information herein, particularly with regard to technique and procedure. However, appropriate informa-tion sources should be consulted, especially for new or unfamiliar procedures. It is the responsibility of every practitioner to evaluate the appropriateness of a particular opinion in the context of actual clinical situations and with due consideration to new developments. Authors, editors, and the publisher cannot be held responsible for any typographical or other errors found in this book.

Editorial Resources: Jane Colilla
Library of Congress Catalog Card Number: 95-14128
ISBN: 0-8342-0622-6

Printed in the United States of America

1     2     3     4     5

# Table of Contents

# Preface

Patients with shoulder pain and dysfunction are increasingly unwilling to modify their life activities to accommodate their symptoms. In the United States and Western Europe, the volume of elective shoulder surgeries and intensive shoulder rehabilitation therapies has risen sharply over the last 5 years. New techniques, both in orthopaedics and physical medicine, have been rapidly introduced and popularized. This technologic flux has often left a gap in understanding among members of different specialties treating the shoulder patient. It is nonetheless essential that the pathophysiology of the major shoulder disorders, rehabilitation issues, and surgical treatment methods be grasped by all members of the health care team.

In physical therapy, a standard treatment plan based on a one-line orthopaedic diagnosis is often inadequate when one is dealing with shoulder patients. For example, with a diagnosis of rotator cuff tear–postrepair, the practitioner in physical medicine may treat a young athlete with an arthroscopically debrided partial-thickness tear. This patient can safely begin resistive cuff strengthening 7 days postoperatively and advance quickly, returning to competition level output at 6 weeks. Carrying the same diagnosis, however, may be a steroid-dependent 65-year-old who had undergone a subscapularis transfer for repair of a massive, ancient tear. This patient risks rerupture of the reconstructed tendons if the shoulder is moved beyond a limited range or if active, eccentric contraction is permitted before 3 months postoperatively.

This book is written for the practitioner in physical medicine and sports medicine as an up-to-date guide to the major elements of modern diagnosis, physical therapy, and surgical treatment. Sports training, rehabilitation, and maintenance therapies are clearly explained with underlying anatomy and pathophysiology. Although the book is written for the professional, parts may be used as a patient resource in explaining rehabilitation issues and surgical procedures.

The book is organized in two main parts. The first explores the general clinical process of problem recognition and orthopaedic work-up, diagnosis, and treatment. This part is a patient-centered overview containing sections on shoulder symptoms, physical examination of the shoulder, radiologic work-up, pharmacologic treatment, the role of physical therapy, and nonmusculoskeletal causes of shoulder pain and dysfunction.

The second part explores each disease area in detail. These chapters are organized according to pathomechanics. Here, and in each subsequent chapter, current understanding of the disease mechanism is presented first so that the rationale of physical and orthopaedic treatments may be fully appreciated. Frozen shoulder, a final common pathway of nearly all shoulder disease, is focused on initially. The wide spectrum of rotator cuff disease is next explored, stressing the subacromial impingement phenomenon. Clinical presentations of this disease range from mild shoulder pain at night to complete joint destruction. Joint instability, from subluxation to frank dislocation, is another major area of shoulder morbidity in the younger patient.

Instability of the acromioclavicular (AC) joint, the other diarthrodial articulation of the shoulder, is addressed in another chapter focused specifically on AC joint disease. Also discussed here is the wide range of clinical problems caused by degeneration of this joint. The contribution of acromioclavicular arthritis to impingement-related disease of the rotator cuff is explained in detail.

The expanding population of active patients with degenerative joint disease of the shoulder represents the challenge discussed in the next chapter. Glenohumeral arthritis arising from trauma, cuff tear, aseptic necrosis of bone, and a variety of primary arthritic processes may be treated conservatively or may require surgical reconstruction with prosthetic replacement of the joint surfaces. Clear understanding of the shoulder replacement procedure, as well as nonsurgical treatments for the arthritic shoulder, are presented. This chapter also includes rehabilitation protocols for patients after the various types of arthroplastic reconstructions.

The shoulder problems of athletes are often the result of a subtle interrelationship of instability and impingement. These are described in a chapter on specific sports medicine problems of the shoulder. Loose bodies in the glenohumeral joint, tears of the glenoid labrum, and biceps tendon syndromes, all associated with complex instability, are discussed. The chapter then goes into sports-oriented rehabilitation as well as technical considerations and the uses and limitations of shoulder arthroscopy.

Because the majority of proximal humerus replacement surgeries are done for patients after complex fractures, this group is discussed in a separate chapter devoted to fractures about the shoulder. Attention in this chapter is given to long-term issues in rehabilitation. Acute fracture care is described for background, although in less detail than in an orthopaedic fracture text.

The final chapter in the book gives the practitioner in physical medicine essential clinical information about a number of less common problems producing shoulder complaints. These include infection, tumor, metabolic disorders, brain diseases, and spinal cord problems that present with shoulder dysfunction and pain.

Although written for a professional audience, this book contains clear and complete explanations of anatomic, biomechanical, and medical terms, making it accessible to students in both physical therapy and medicine. The book has been prepared as a guide to treatment, but care has been taken to avoid giving the professional simplified recipes or protocols for treatment to be applied on the basis of a supplied diagnosis. Instead, the entire diagnostic process is examined with evaluation from orthopaedic, physiatric, and radiologic points of view. The broad range of modern shoulder therapeutics is then explained in light of current pathophysiologic understanding. In this elucidation of treatment lies the work's ultimate goal: intelligent participation in treatment decisions with more meaningful and effective involvement in the shoulder patient's care. It should provide a scholarly yet practical reference.

# Acknowledgments

Heartfelt thanks and a student's debt of gratitude are expressed to Charles S. Neer II, who taught me and so many others how to think clearly about the shoulder.

My admiration and deep gratitude are also expressed to Louis U. Bigliani and Evan Flatow of the New York Orthopedic Hospital for their friendship and teaching in the area of shoulder surgery. Charles Rockwood, a frequent Visiting Professor at Columbia, has also been a great teacher of the shoulder to me, as has his student Wayne Burkhead.

Harold M. Dick, Chief of the Orthopaedic Service at the Columbia Presbyterian Medical Center, has been an inspiration as a leader of great intelligence and character to all of us who have served as his residents. Christopher B. Michelsen of the New York Orthopedic Hospital has similarly been a friend of consistent character and superb technical skills in surgery.

Finally, two of my greatest mentors in orthopaedics and life have been A.C. Haig and the late Frank E. Stinchfield. Their lessons of integrity and persistence continue to guide me.

# Part I

# Modern Shoulder Practice

# Chapter 1

# Symptomatology

This book is about shoulder problems: what they are and how they can be successfully treated. The anticipated reader will be involved with the diagnosis, treatment, and rehabilitation of shoulder problems in physical medicine and sports medicine. The shoulder is one of the fastest growing areas within orthopaedics today. There are many new procedures and much new understanding of joint pathophysiology. Clear explanation of current practices in shoulder treatment, both surgical and nonsurgical, is one goal of this book.

The shoulder is certainly the most complex joint in the body. Its normal range of motion is greater and can be expressed in more directions than that of any other joint. Many of its ailments, including the most common ones, involve biomechanical mechanisms that are unique to the shoulder. Therapy relies heavily on exercises done in specific positions of the joint because intra- and extraarticular structures move simultaneously with every motion of the scapula on the thorax and of the humerus on the scapula. Although the great majority of shoulder patients are successfully treated without surgery (about 80% in the author's practice), patients treated with an operation, even an arthroscopic one, have a greater reliance on postoperative physical treatment than nonsurgical patients.

An extraordinarily high level of communication is necessary among the shoulder patient, therapist, and orthopaedist for accurate diagnosis and effective treatment. This book hopes to facilitate this by creating a common understanding of the diagnostic and therapeutic techniques used by all members of the health care team. A shoulder problem can be merely nagging, or it can completely destroy the quality of a person's life. Good understanding of the pertinent pathophysiology and all aspects of therapeutics is soon communicated to one's patients. This communication often becomes an important step toward cure.

Athletes with shoulder pain, particularly tennis players, golfers, baseball or softball players, and weightlifters are singled out in many sections of the book. Serious participation in sport is a wonderful enrichment of many patients' lives. Athletes place greater demands on their shoulders than nonathletes and often bring out symptoms of an underlying shoulder condition that might otherwise have gone unnoticed. When an avid tennis player asks "Is my shoulder pain caused by tennis?" he or she usually knows the answer. A difference between traditional medicine and sports medicine is demonstrated by this. Thirty years ago an orthopaedist might simply have treated this patient with the prescription "no more tennis." Today, the option of therapy and even surgery to maintain comfortable athletic performance is given to many patients who are far from being professional athletes. Much current day shoulder practice falls into this sports medicine category, even in older patients. It is therefore not unusual to provide treatment for shoulder pain that is purely sports related. Familiarity with the specific demands placed on the shoulder by various sports is therefore essential for many practitioners today. Athletes of any age are generally good patients and get good results because they are interested and motivated. Much of what is said about them is applicable to all shoulder patients.

## PAIN PATTERNS AND PAIN HISTORY

Establishing a diagnosis for many shoulder problems can be quite difficult. Symptom complexes overlap and findings on physical examination may be inconsistent. Overly sensitive tests such as magnetic resonance imaging can confuse the diagnosis because the pathology seen on the test may not be responsible for the presenting symptoms. Accurate diagnosis is certainly a necessary step toward successful treatment of shoulder pathology. Although diagnosis is commonly perceived as purely a physician's responsibility, concerned practitioners at every station—physician, surgeon, therapist, nurse, or physiatrist—should think diagnostically, examining and reexamining the data a patient presents at each contact. Typical presentations of most common problems are usually discernible in the patient's history.

When a new patient is treated, the following questions should be asked:

- Problem definition
  1. Where does it hurt?
  2. Can you place one fingertip where the pain is worst?

3. When does it hurt?
4. Does it hurt right now?
5. Does it hurt at night?
6. What positions make it worse?
7. What activities make it worse?
8. Is there pain with overhead work?
9. Does exercise make it worse?
10. Is it worse the next day after exercise?
11. What specific exercise seems to cause the most problem?
12. For how long has it hurt?
13. Is it more severe than usual now?

- Characterization
    1. What is the pain like?
    2. Is there associated numbness of the hand or arm?
    3. Does the pain remind you of a similar past episode?
    4. Are there movements you just can't perform any longer?
    5. Are there movements that are particularly weak?
    6. Does the shoulder "come out of joint"?
    7. Does the arm "go dead"?
    8. Is there a catching sensation?

- Background
    1. Do you have any history of significant medical illness, specifically diabetes, heart disease, lung disease, arthritic disease, or nervous system disease?
    2. Do you have any history of dislocation, fracture, surgery, or injury to the shoulder?

The answers to these questions are usually sufficient to direct the practitioner to the correct general area of diagnosis. These initial data are best reviewed and the questions asked again at later visits; the answers often change. The examiner must sift through any data that are in conflict for the dominant features of the pain. Most basically, the data necessary to start the diagnostic investigation are the pain's location and temporal pattern. The following section deals with general diagnostic patterns. These are used to organize the practitioner's approach to the initial diagnosis of the shoulder problem. Significantly greater detail is found in the chapters on individual disease areas in the second part of this book.

## DIAGNOSTIC PATTERNS: PAIN LOCATION

### Neck

Neck pain is frequently caused by shoulder pathology. Although many practitioners are familiar with the referral of pain along dermatomal or myotomal routes, such patterns are usually considered in distal radiation only. This is to say that pain felt distal to a pathologic locus is the expected referral pattern. A common exception to this is found with irritation in the subacromial area.

*Subacromial cervicalgia* is the term used to describe pain whose origin is mechanical irritation in the space below the acromion but is felt in the neck, parascapular area, trapezius area, and even occasionally into the side of the head with associated tinnitus (ringing in the ears).[1] This type of pain is usually worse when the arm is overhead and is described as shooting or sharp. It is most commonly felt in the trapezius area and base of neck (Figure 1–1). There is occasionally nothing but neck or upper back pain, with nothing at all to suggest a shoulder origin.

It is certainly true that many purely cervical problems produce neck pain. Arthritis, disc herniation or degeneration, and cervical muscle injury or spasm

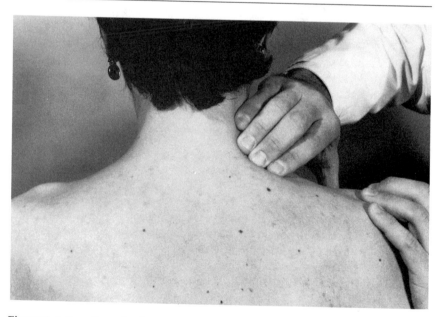

**Figure 1–1** Location of pain: subacromial cervicalgia.

are examples. Pain produced by localized pressure on the cervical nerve roots is often of an electrical or shooting nature and is associated with numbness or weakness in the arm. Patients with these pains also will recognize their clear relationship to certain positions of the neck and not to neck motion in general. The historical distinction between these and subacromial cervicalgia is subtle but discernible; both types of patients will complain of pain while driving. The true neck pain patient will complain most about backing up and having to turn the neck, whereas the subacromial cervicalgia patient will have increased neck pain with long periods of holding the wheel with the shoulders flexed. Neck patients usually get some relief from taking the weight of the head off the neck, such as when lying down flat. Subacromial cervicalgia patients often have increased neck pain in bed at night because greater impingement tends to occur when the humerus is not being pulled down vertically by gravity. The diagnosis of subacromial cervicalgia is made by physical examination and injection test. Questioning the patient along the lines of the examination is usually revealing, however. Overhead activity typically increases the pain of subacromial cervicalgia; this position is similar to the impingement test used to diagnose the problem.

A frequently confounding problem occurs when both phenomena, cervical spine disease and subacromial cervicalgia, simultaneously contribute to symptomatology. This is not unusual because cervical arthrosis, disc degeneration, and disc herniation are so common. Physical examination and injection testing are then necessary to elucidate which is the dominant pathology.

### Acromioclavicular Joint Area

Pain felt specifically in the acromioclavicular (AC) joint is often simply due to arthritis of that joint. On questioning of the patient, the pain will be seen to be worst when the arm is used across the body horizontally, such as when washing the contralateral axilla. Patients often volunteer to demonstrate the tender, bony bump on top of their shoulder. They should be asked if finger pressure on the bump (the AC joint; Figure 1–2) produces pain of similar character to their presenting complaint. Although physical examination, X-rays, and sometimes an injection test are needed to make this diagnosis, the historical findings of an enlarging, tender, bony bump on the shoulder with night pain from sleeping on the painful side and pain when placing the arm across the body are in themselves highly suggestive of AC joint pain. Patients involved in weight training often develop this problem; it first becomes symptomatic with bench and military press.

Pain that patients describe as being felt primarily 2 cm or so below the AC joint inside the shoulder is often due to tearing or fraying of the glenoid labrum (see Figure 1–2). Cartilaginous loss (arthrosis) or a fracture of the glenoid rim may also produce this pattern of pain. These are often "catching" pains that are felt intermittently when the arm is rotated around the long axis of the humerus in certain degrees of abduction. Catching pain at this subclavicular location is likely to present in the shoulder-intensive athlete. This patient often complains that the pain only becomes intense when throwing, serving the tennis ball, or hurling the javelin. On questioning, it is often apparent that a certain part of the throwing motion brings on the pain. The differential diagnosis is rather broad for throwing-specific pain felt just under the AC joint, but the structures of the anterior glenohumeral joint should be placed under consideration. This is not a location to which the pain of distant pathology often refers or radiates.

### Subacromial Area

The acromial process of the scapula is the flat bone at the point of the shoulder. Pain felt just under the front edge of this flat bone (Figure 1–3) is typical of

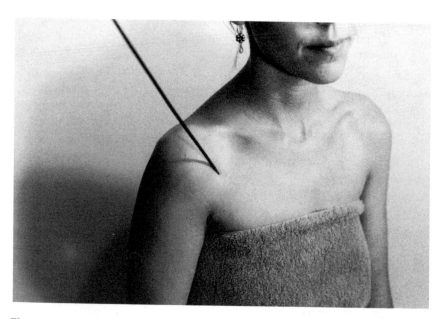

**Figure 1–2** Location of pain: AC joint disease and anterior glenohumeral joint pain.

impingement syndrome and rotator cuff tear. The pain is worse when the arm is raised straight overhead. It is momentarily sharp when the arm is overhead and then becomes a strong aching after the arm is brought down. Some patients also describe a jamming pain when the arm is high; this is an accurate description of what is actually going on at the subacromial interval.

Subacromial pain that is felt to be maximal at a location about 2 cm or so medial to the midbody of the acromion (see Figure 1–3C) is frequently the chief symptom of bicipital tendinitis. It is important that the patient be as specific as possible in pointing out the location of greatest pain, but with careful questioning it can often be established that the pain is not localized to the AC joint and is not of the deep anterior nature that anterior capsular or glenoid pathology produces. This patient is also likely to volunteer a physical examination sign: tenderness at this point. Bicipital tendinitis pain also typically radiates into the anterior arm. Patients will complain of pain anteriorly in the arm with activities such as forceful gripping and turning a screwdriver.

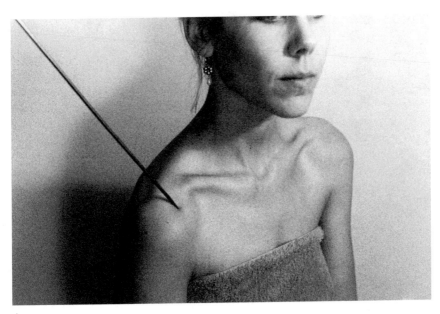

**A**

**Figure 1–3 (A)** Location of the subacromial area, often tender in cases of rotator cuff tendinitis or chronic impingement.

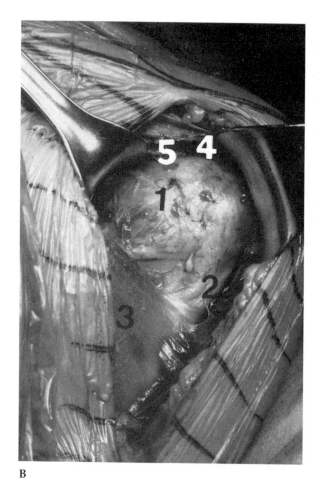

**B**

**Figure 1–3 (B)** Surgical exposure of the left anterior shoulder; the deltoid is retracted to the patient's left, the pectoralis major to the right. 1, subscapularis tendon; 2, biceps long head tendon; 3, pectoralis major; 4, subacromial space; 5, coracoacromial ligament.

## Posterior Shoulder

The posterior aspect of the glenohumeral joint is palpable 2 cm below and 2 cm medial to the posterior acromial angle; see Figure 1–4 and Chapter 2 for accurate localization of these landmarks. Many patients with anterior instability complain of sharp, intermittent pain at the posterior joint line during maneuvers that permit significant anterior translation of the humeral head on the

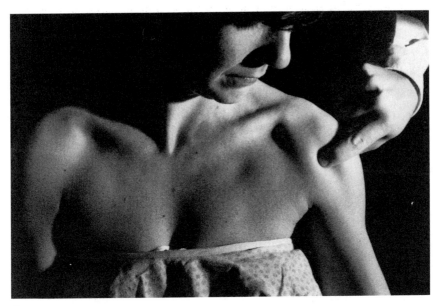

C

**Figure 1–3 (C)** Palpation of the bicipital groove between the greater and lesser tuberosities. Surface anatomy of the strap muscles (biceps short head and coracobrachialis) is visible just media to the examiner's fingertip.

glenoid. Historical details from such patients with anterior instability are likely to include episodes of "dead arm" while playing at sports; this constitutes a short period during which the entire arm is numb and powerless. There may have been frank dislocations or the feeling that the shoulder is about to dislocate when it is in certain positions. When a patient localizes pain to the posterior shoulder, he or she may be describing the posterior deltoid, the latissimus dorsi, or even the periscapular muscles. Most people can distinguish these muscular pains, which are common, from the sharper and deeper joint pain that occurs with instability. Patients should be asked if it feel muscular in nature.

A specific posterior shoulder pain is felt by some athletes during posterior loading of the joint with bench press and push-ups. This is catching and intermittent, usually stopping immediately when pressure is let off the joint. It is commonly of sufficient severity to make the athlete stop doing these exercises completely. Posterior glenoid labral tears often start at the part of the labrum associated with the insertion of the biceps tendon (this is termed a SLAP lesion and is discussed in Chapter 9). These tears frequently are responsible for this

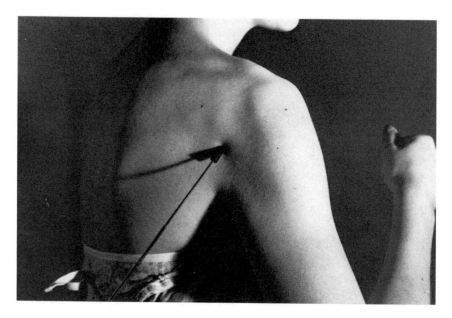

**Figure 1–4** Posterior glenohumeral joint area. Tenderness here is associated with glenohumeral synovitis and arthritis.

symptom. It is unfortunately true that posterior joint line pain in the young shoulder patient may result from both anterior and posterior glenohumeral joint instability and the capsular and labral damage that this produces. It remains for the physical examination to determine the direction or directions of the instability.

A completely different diagnosis produces the complaint of posterior shoulder pain in most older patients who are not involved in athletics. Glenohumeral arthritis and adhesive capsulitis both may cause a patient to indicate that the greatest pain is at the posterior aspect of the glenohumeral joint. Because they are frequently concomitant, frozen shoulder and glenohumeral arthritis should be separated historically and must be clearly distinct to the practitioner.

"I can't move my arm normally" is a frequent complaint among shoulder patients. The history of increasing shoulder pain for years, a grinding, catching, and even squeaking with joint motion, loss of range of motion, and finally worsening pain felt in the posterior aspect of the joint with any motion of the arm strongly suggest arthritis of the glenohumeral joint. Arthritis in the shoulder, as elsewhere, produces an aching pain that may respond to antiinflammatory drugs. Adhesive capsulitis, or frozen shoulder, produces soreness everywhere around the shoulder. The pain is felt primarily at the ends of range of motion. The patient may complain mostly of posterior joint line pain but usually will be found to be most hampered by loss of range and will admit to nearly as much pain anteriorly on questioning.

### Deltoid Insertion Area and Upper Arm

A common location of pain in patients with rotator cuff impingement, this area is vaguely described by most patients who have pain here. They often grab the fleshy part of the upper arm (Figure 1–5) and complain of a deep pain in the muscle. Their problem is almost never in the muscle, however, but rather in the tendons of the rotator cuff underneath the acromion. Pain at the deltoid insertion area is common and almost completely nonspecific as a diagnostic indicator because nearly any shoulder problem can cause rotator cuff irritation. An accompanying history of direct trauma to the shoulder area or intense training involving deltoid isolation exercise suggests the possibility of actual deltoid insertional pain (ie, deltoid tendon strain or tendinitis). This is

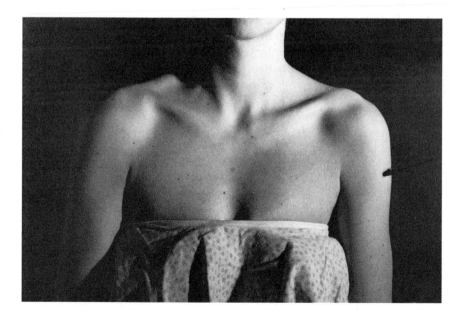

**Figure 1–5** Deltoid insertion area. This is commonly the location of pain associated with rotator cuff disease.

rare but not difficult to diagnose because it does produce local tenderness at the deltoid insertion, whereas none of the rotator cuff–related problems does so.

The practitioner should note the mysterious tendency for the three flat tendons that form a hood over the humeral head to produce pain somewhere else when they are irritated. Damage and inflammation of the cuff may produce pain high in the neck, in the trapezius, under the acromion (where the problem actually is), at the deltoid insertion, and occasionally just above the elbow. The capacity accurately to localize pain signals from the rotator cuff tendons is poor in most people. This is one reason why few shoulder patients present with an accurate idea of what is wrong with their shoulder.

### Scapula

The rhomboids—small, flat, squarish muscles that attach to the medial border of the scapula—are often tender and spastic after an acute shoulder injury (Figure 1–6). These muscles retract and rotate the scapula. They absorb much energy in eccentric contraction during motions requiring rapid scapular protraction. Throwers are especially apt to complain of pain in the rhomboid area after a heavy workout early in their season. The muscles are tender in these patients, and there may be a history of favorable response to massage or liniment application. The pain is definitely muscular in character, although rather sharp. Pain at the medial scapular border may also be associated with whiplash injuries of the neck. The patient should be questioned regarding neck injuries if medial scapular pain is the presenting complaint. Scapulothoracic bursitis may also produce pain at this location. There will generally be a report of a grating sensation with scapular motion on the thorax. Historical detail is usually insufficient to separate scapular rotator pain from scapulothoracic articular pain.

### Chest

Chest pain, even if felt high in the chest or under the clavicle, is far more likely to be of cardiac origin than related to a shoulder problem. Cardiac pain may radiate to the jaw or down one or both arms or may stay in the chest. Obviously, questioning about cardiac history is necessary if any history of chest pain is given. Cardiac pain is usually unaffected by position of the arm or use of the shoulder girdle muscles. Rib, abdominal, and chest wall muscle pathology may produce chest pains as well; a history of much coughing, direct trauma to the chest, or tender spots on the chest wall tend to suggest this type of noncardiac chest pain.

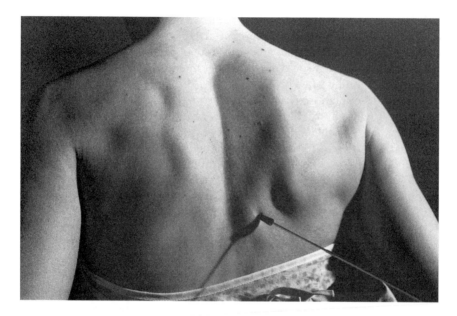

**Figure 1–6** Rhomboid muscles, surface anatomy.

## GLOBAL, ACUTE, AND SEVERE SHOULDER PAIN

Although nervous patients in pain tend to say that their pain is everywhere, once they have been calmed down and questioned they can usually be specific about a particular focus. Some shoulder problems are marked by pain and tenderness all around the shoulder with little difference in perceived pain from front to back or side to side. The pain is diffuse and worsens with just about any motion. The most worrisome condition to present this way is infection. Septic arthritis of the glenohumeral joint is due to bacterial infection. The joint is a particularly dangerous place for infection because it contains potential spaces that are outside the reach of the immune system cells that normally assist in ridding the body of bacterial invaders. Septic arthritis can occur with gonorrhea, sickle cell disease, intravenous drug use, acquired immunodeficiency syndrome (AIDS), other immunosuppressed states such as disseminated cancer or chemotherapy, and bacterial endocarditis. The diagnosis is suggested by historical details that include any of these plus a history of fevers, chills, weight loss, increasing malaise, and increasing pain. The diagnosis must be secured by putting a needle into the joint and getting out pus. The patient with a septic shoulder can be recognized in most cases because he or she is clearly sick.

Nearly as painful, although somewhat less dangerous, is the shoulder with acute calcium deposits in the rotator cuff. Unlike the case of septic shoulder, there is a location of maximal tenderness about which the patient may complain. The pain is often so severe, however, that the complaint that the entire shoulder is painful is often given.

Acute, severe shoulder pain and diffuse glenohumeral tenderness may occur (rarely) with gouty arthritis. This disease is much more common in the peripheral joints of the feet and hands, but it can occur in the shoulder. The presentation is similar to that of infection, with diffuse, terrible pain, tenderness, and fever. The patient will probably not be difficult to diagnose because shoulder attacks of gout occur almost exclusively in patients with established gouty disease. Most of these patients will be able to recognize all too readily that they are having another gouty attack.

A milder version of the acute calcium deposit presentation is seen in some cases of bicipital tendinitis. As mentioned earlier, this pain is usually felt anteriorly, somewhere below the acromion. It can be so intense as to merit the "everywhere" designation. Pain may also be dramatically increased with nearly any motion of the arm or shoulder in cases of severe bicipital tendinitis.

The early phases of adhesive capsulitis are associated with pain around the entire shoulder girdle. Although the pain is not typically as severe as that associated with septic shoulder and calcific tendinitis, it is diffuse and associated with global tenderness. The complaints from this patient center more about loss of shoulder motion as the early, inflammatory phase of this problem subsides, leaving the shoulder capsule stuck to itself and the humeral head.

## SYMPTOM COMPLEXES IN COMMON DISORDERS

### Rotator Cuff Disease and Impingement

The diagnostic history is naturally broken down into pain localization (what hurts?) and pain patterns (when does it hurt?). These patterns are among the least specific clues to diagnosis by themselves because there is so much symptom overlap among different disorders. The examiner should be sensitive to pain patterns, however, because they are usually what start him or her thinking about the right diagnosis. The most useful pain patterns to look for when one is considering rotator cuff disease, for a first example, are night pain and pain with overhead work. Night pain is described by some as an inability to find a comfortable position for the arm. Overhead work pain, such as pain with putting dishes away on high shelves, may be in the shoulder or trapezius and neck. Patients often will admit to sleeping in an easy chair to prevent the night pain. Recognizing this pattern in the initial history, the examiner is prompted both to ask more specific questions about impingement-related pain and to examine more carefully for signs of rotator cuff disease and impingement.

Younger patients with rotator cuff disease usually have sports-related pain that increases with overhand throwing, shooting a basketball, and serving in tennis (especially the topspun twist serve and hard, flat serves). Night pain and overhead pain with normal living activities are less of an issue. Determined baseball and softball players may give the history of having switched to sidearm throwing to avoid the pain. A sore shoulder after a serving or pitching workout is typical in a young rotator cuff patient's story.

**Glenohumeral Instability**

The unstable shoulder is much less commonly a problem in the older population than in younger, active patients. As with rotator cuff patients, serving and throwing are apt to be painful. The symptom complex seen with impingers, however, includes pain that lasts for hours to days after hard overhead use, whereas the pain with instability tends to disappear rapidly. Of course, the history of true shoulder dislocation on the symptomatic side makes the diagnosis of instability quite likely. Instability patients have trouble when the arm is abducted and externally rotated, especially if any force is applied in a posterior direction while in this position. The arm may "go dead," becoming numb and weak for a few seconds after trauma in the abducted, externally rotated position. As instability becomes more severe, it becomes easier to diagnose because the patient is more likely to complain that the shoulder feels as if it is sloppier or about to go out of joint. Instability pain may be felt anteriorly or posteriorly; it is usually sharp, intermittent, and highly positional. Except in the case of severe subluxation or true dislocation, it is likely not to be worse the day after. Pain that is worse the next day suggests muscular or rotator cuff etiology.

**Arthritis**

Arthritic pain, in general, tends to be worse in the morning or after a period of inactivity. The pain tends to decrease somewhat after the joint and its surrounding tissues are warmed up by activity. This is more likely to be true for osteoarthritic or posttraumatic arthritic pain than for inflammatory arthritic (eg, rheumatoid) pain. Classically, the rheumatoid patient feels best in the morning and gets progressively worse during the day. Shoulder arthritis is usually accompanied by progressive loss of motion, which may be a large part of the presenting symptom complex. Arthritis shoulder pain tends to be helped more by antiinflammatory drugs, such as aspirin, than any other type of shoulder pain. Impingement pain is helped to some small extent; instability pain is hardly ever improved by these drugs. The warmth of a shower often brings welcome relief to arthritic shoulders, and weather ache, felt especially on cold, damp days, is often a prominent feature.

AC joint arthritis produces positional shoulder pain that is usually worst in bed when the patient is lying on the side. Arm motions across the body, such as when putting up the hair or washing the opposite axilla, are painful early in the course of the disease. As the arthritic changes of the joint become more severe, pain patterns that mimic those of impingement are seen. Overhead pain, night pain, and pain with keeping the arms horizontal (as with driving) become prominent. The younger patient with AC pain is likely to be a weightlifter or to have a history of distal clavicular fracture. The first weight-lifting exercise to become painful is often the bench or military press. AC pain is helped by antiinflammatory agents. The history of increased pain from the pressure of shoulder straps (such as those on camera bags, luggage, or even a purse) is likely to indicate AC arthritis.

### Loose Intraarticular Bodies

Tears of the glenoid labrum or loose bony or cartilaginous bodies in the glenohumeral joint produce the symptom of a sharp, sudden pain that is felt in a certain position, but not always the same one. The pain usually goes away suddenly with a small movement of the shoulder. This is most common in throwing athletes (curve ball pitchers) and painters (of houses). Weightlifters have subtle instabilities that may present with symptomatic loose bodies or labral tear pain. Flies and reverse flies tend to bring out these symptoms, especially while the weight is being lowered.

### Shoulder Fractures and Sudden Tears

A common pattern of pain is marked by an injury, fall, or accident that seems to have started the entire problem. Pain that starts with an injury is often caused by a fracture. A rotator cuff tear may also occur suddenly with an injury. The pain from this may not be severe, but the loss of power will be noticed immediately. These acute tears may not be related to the impingement phenomenon but rather to poor vascularity of the rotator cuff and its increasing stiffness with age. One of the two heads (the long head) of the biceps muscle may also rupture suddenly, without any preexisting symptoms, during an accidental fall or other forceful use of the arm. This produces some pain and bruising, but most telling is the painless lump that suddenly appears in the anterior aspect of the arm.

## RELATIVE FREQUENCIES OF THE SHOULDER DISORDERS

Although the clinician should keep his or her mind open for any possibility, it is good practice to maintain an appreciation for the frequencies with which the common, electively treated shoulder ailments occur. Knowing the rough statistical likelihood of a given problem tends to sharpen one's diagnostic acumen. Although it is not possible to establish scientifically, the most common shoulder pain is most likely to be caused by mild overuse of the shoulder girdle muscles, particularly the rotator cuff. The patient with mild, transient pain generally does not seek professional help and therefore this is conjecture, but overuse pain occurs so frequently in the course of shoulder rehabilitation that it is probably equally frequent in the untreated population (Table 1–1).

In the community orthopaedic shoulder surgeon's practice, the most common problem is definitely impingement syndrome with or without rotator cuff tear. This makes up approximately 40% of shoulder referrals. AC joint disorders are also quite common (about 15%). Instability, free bodies, and labral tears, taken together, represent roughly 25% of presentations, and glenohumeral arthritis is diagnosed in about 5% of cases. Biceps tendinitis, pure frozen shoulder without an underlying cause, calcific tendinitis, and pure trapezius spasm without underlying cause represent about 10% of cases, which leaves tumors, infections, congenital defects, and nervous system and circulatory problems for the remaining 5%.

It is of course ridiculous to use statistical occurrence as a diagnostic aid. These frequencies are apt to be different in the practice of physical therapists, medical sports medicine practitioners, and university-based surgeons. The average age of the patients in a practice will also influence these frequencies.

---

**Table 1–1** Shoulder Pain: Rough Frequencies of Diagnosis in Author's Community Practice

| | |
|---|---|
| Impingement and Rotator Cuff Disease | 40% |
| Instability and Related Disorders | 25% |
| Acromioclavicular Joint Disorders | 15% |
| Frozen Shoulder, Tendinitis, and Overuse | 10% |
| Glenohumeral Arthritis | 5% |
| Other Shoulder Diagnoses | 5% |

They are best used for comparison and as a self-checking device for one's diagnostic ability. The practitioner who finds himself or herself discovering a fourth case of septic glenohumeral arthritis that morning should question his or her accuracy in shoulder diagnosis.

---

**REFERENCE**

1. Michelsen C. Personal communication, 1986.

# Chapter 2

# Physical Examination of the Shoulder

## PERFORMING THE EXAMINATION

Repeated physical examination of the shoulder is the single most important diagnostic tool available to the practitioner. Findings on physical examination should be recorded carefully because they often change. In a confusing or difficult diagnostic situation, the correct diagnosis is often the one supported by the majority of the physical findings the majority of the time. The therapist, physiatrist, and surgeon have the physical examination as common ground, and it is not at all infrequent that the careful physical findings of a student therapist lead to the correct diagnosis and treatment plan, which may have eluded the senior members of the team. Inherent here is a caution against overreliance on radiographic studies: If the magnetic resonance image says impingement but the physical examination shows only acromioclavicular (AC) joint signs, it is generally prudent to treat only the AC joint.

General appearance, including habitus (endomorphic, mesomorphic, or ectomorphic), gait abnormalities, posture, and affect, is recorded on initial examination. Although avoiding premature formulations based on these external appearances, the discriminating practitioner may use these data to advantage in coming to a diagnosis. For example, if a thin, sickly, pale patient with a racking cough, sunken eyes, and needle tracks on the arms complains of intense shoulder pain, septic arthritis should be considered immediately. The patient with a marfanoid habitus (a gangly ectomorph) is likely to have hyperligamentous laxity and pain related to joint instability. The tests for hyperligamentous laxity include thumb to forearm, in which the patient is asked to try to touch the thumb to the ipsilateral forearm (the result being recorded as positive if he or she can; Figure 2–1). The ability to hyperextend the elbows beyond 5° is also considered by many to indicate a tendency toward hyperligamentous laxity.

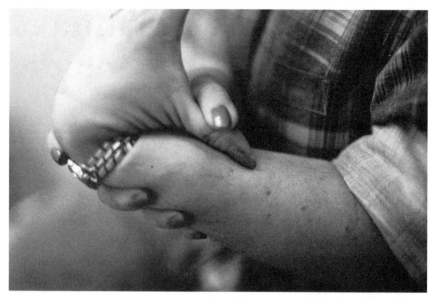

A

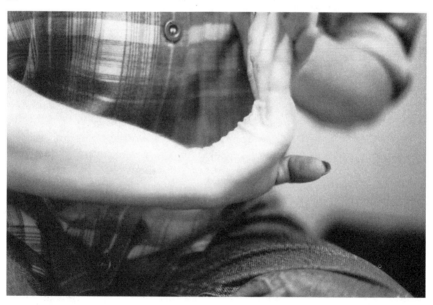

B

**Figure 2–1** Tests of hyperligamentous laxity. **(A)** Thumb-to-forearm and **(B)** metacarpophalangeal joint hyperextension.

Gait abnormalities often indicate neurologic abnormalities. The shu gait of Parkinson's disease in a shoulder patient is frequently associated v ..a simple adhesive capsulitis. Parkinson's disease, diabetes mellitus (probably working through its associated neuropathy), and cerebrovascular accidents are among the more common neurologic disorders that are associated with a high incidence of idiopathic adhesive capsulitis.

Regarding the patient with unusual affect, it is important not to let one's personal reaction to the patient cloud the simple processes of reason used in diagnosis. It is woefully true that a great percentage of patients today experience a greater degree of pain and dysfunction than they would otherwise because, wittingly or not, they are programming themselves to perform a legal charade for which they expect to be paid much money. An examiner's suspicion of this should be recorded in the most objective terms possible. There are, nonetheless, many other causes of unusual behavior, two of which are fear and pain. An important tool for use in the physical examination is therefore the social skill (perhaps grace) used to relax the patient sufficiently to permit a good examination.

Posture should be observed in the shoulder patient, especially in patients with muscular complaints about the shoulder girdle, neck, and upper back. The presence of an increased thoracic kyphosis (Figure 2–2) with a compensatory increase in cervical lordosis is commonly seen in patients with "droopy" shoulders who complain of trapezius and upper back pain along the medial scapular borders. Chronically bad posture or occupational postural demands that force patients to lean forward with the arms outstretched for long periods produce the same type of increased myofascial tension in the scapular positioning muscles. Seated posture, especially at a computer keyboard, is another frequent cause of mild muscular pain about the shoulder girdle. This is easily simulated during the examination.

Downsloping, chronically protracted scapulae are also felt, by some orthopaedists, to be related to posterior glenohumeral (GH) instability. The possibility of the posterior capsule becoming stretched and the glenoid tending to slip forward on the humeral head in this situation is plausible but has not been established from observations at surgery. It is good to pay attention to the carriage of the shoulder girdles as well as the spinal posture in the physical examination. Special attention to the GH instability examination is also warranted if postural findings such as these are present.

## NECK

The neck is usually examined first when a shoulder examination is performed. With the patient seated, the neck is palpated from behind for masses,

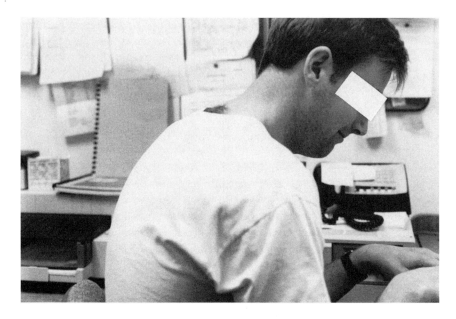

**Figure 2–2**  Increased thoracic kyphosis and "droopy" shoulders.

enlargement of the thyroid, muscular symmetry, muscular tenderness, and bony tenderness at the mastoids, occiput, and posterior spinous processes. The patient is asked to rotate the neck maximally left and right and then to flex (put the chin on the chest) and extend (put the head back as far as possible) the neck, with range of motion in degrees being recorded for each of these four movements. A patient with pain during the examination is asked which maneuver increases the pain most and which, if any, decreases it. The head is firmly pushed straight down from the crown, and then gentle axial traction is applied, again with questioning for the effect of these maneuvers on the type, location, and severity of pain (Figure 2–3). Side-to-side tilt and finally the effect on pain of gently assisted extension with tilt to each side are recorded.

Many shoulder patients have neck pain, and it is the first purpose of this examination to establish the presence or absence of any intrinsic neck problem that may be responsible for the patient's symptoms. Extension-tilt and axial loading typically increase the pain of cervical nerve root compression, and axial traction typically relieves it. The neck pain of subacromial cervicalgia (see Chapter 8) typically is increased by attempted rotation but not by flexion and extension. The examination of the neck should always be slow and gentle, avoiding pressure on the carotid arteries and with attention to any symptoms,

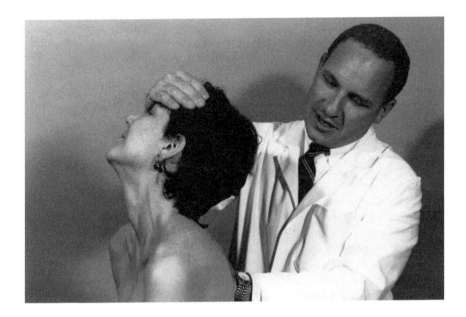

**Figure 2–3** Extension-tilt of the neck.

such as pain, tingling, or numbness in the neck, back, and arms, that are elicited on the examining maneuver.

## NEUROLOGIC

The neurologic examination of the shoulder patient may be done rapidly as part of muscle testing, with sensory and reflex responses being checked as the arms and forearms are examined. The neurologic examination is focused initially on screening for gross abnormalities or possible neurologic causes for the patient's complaint. It can become detailed and time consuming in cases of subtle central lesions, early presentations of degenerative neurologic or neuromuscular disease, or even the less common entrapment neuropathies. Herein presented, therefore, is the basic neurologic screen through which shoulder patients are put. Further specifics are described in the individual disease chapters.

Note at first the patient's mental status—whether he or she is alert or confused and oriented or disoriented to person, place, and time—and whether his or her affect is appropriate to the content of discussion and the maneuvers through which he or she is being put. Next, gait abnormalities and habitus are important neurologically; a bit of rotator cuff weakness in the 80-year-old, 90-pound woman who comes in using a walker is probably not as significant neurologically as in the 190-pound discus thrower, in whom it may mean suprascapular nerve entrapment.

Check cutaneous light touch sensation along all surfaces of the upper extremities, specifically the hands. Motor function of the arm and forearm muscles is checked by noting strength in fanning the fingers, making a fist, dorsiflexing and volar flexing the wrists, flexing and extending the elbows, and pronating and supinating the forearms. Check finally for the peripheral nerve problems that can produce shoulder symptoms. These include thoracic outlet, anterior scalene, or scapular notch entrapment, brachial plexopathy, and Pancoast's tumors. Tenderness at the lateral aspect of the base of the neck is nonspecific, but this is the location of the brachial plexus. The plexus is especially likely to be under compression if pressure here produces a radiation of pain or paresthesia into the arm or hand. The pressure may be applied by a cervical rib or prominent anterior scalene muscle. These are cases of thoracic outlet syndrome, which occasionally presents with pain around the shoulder. The Adson test is performed to evaluate for this. Here, the neck is turned toward the affected shoulder, and the shoulder is horizontally abducted both to increase pain and paresthesia and to decrease the radial pulse.

The scapular notch (Figure 2–4) is about 4 cm medial to the AC joint and about 2 cm posterior to the clavicle. The suprascapular nerve runs through it to the supraspinatus and infraspinatus muscles. Extreme tenderness at this location is seen in cases of chronic entrapment. Rotator cuff weakness in the absence of impingement should alert one to the possibility of this condition. Palpate gently because the pain produced is intense enough to produce vasovagal reactions, including fainting, when the entrapment is severe.

The Pancoast tumor is any tumor at the dome of the pleura.[1] A tumor at this location may press on the neurologic structures immediately above. Local tenderness and fullness under the midclavicle are sometimes seen with this, in addition to ulnar or low plexus distribution pain and paresthesia. The classic presentation also includes loss of sympathetic tone to the ipsilateral face or Horner's syndrome (dry eye, droopy lid, and constricted pupil).

## SHOULDER GIRDLE

### The Sternoclavicular Joint

The sternoclavicular joint is palpated from behind when the neck examination is completed. Check here for symmetry, tenderness, and size (Figure 2–5).

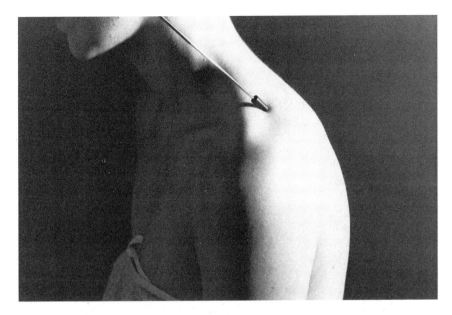

A

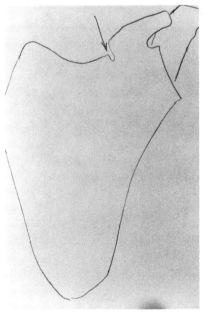

B

**Figure 2–4** Location of the scapular notch.

The sternoclavicular joint is not commonly a source of much pain. It can, however, be dislocated or subluxated after trauma, and if the direction of dislocation is posterior, it can dangerously compress the large blood vessels immediately behind it. If significant asymmetry is detected, it is essential to check the circulatory status of both upper extremities for presence and quality of brachial and radial pulses and venous engorgement.

The sternoclavicular joints are the two bony knobs on either side of the jugular notch. By rasping the medial clavicles (in patients who are neither very fat nor very muscular), the examiner can assess stability of the joints. There is normally little motion possible here. Old trauma and rheumatoid arthritis are most often responsible for any detectable instability, although it is rarely symptomatic. Sternoclavicular arthritis is common, but it, too, is rarely the cause of much pain. When it is, the joint is enlarged and reproducibly tender to palpation. The pain produced by the examination is also the same pain of which the patient complains. It is good practice to ask "Is this like the pain you've been having?" whenever one is palpating a tender area.

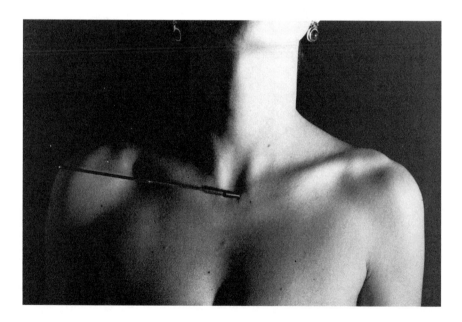

**Figure 2–5** Sternoclavicular joint.

**AC Joint**

The AC joint is palpated next, again from behind the patient, after walking the fingers out along the clavicles from the sternoclavicular joints. The AC joints vary tremendously in size; in many patients they can be spotted from across the room, whereas in others they are hard to locate with careful palpation. They are checked for tenderness and relative size first. An increase in either of these is a sign of arthritis of the joint. The horizontal adduction test (Figure 2–6), more commonly termed the AC grind test, is then done. Here, the arm is adducted or brought across the body in the horizontal plane at shoulder height or slightly below. This produces the same type of pain as palpation of the AC joint in patients with AC arthritis. This test is not diagnostic of AC arthritis, however. Most patients with high-grade impingement alone have some pain with this maneuver. This pain will be eliminated in these impingers with a subacromial injection of local anesthetic. True AC joint pain will only be relieved with anesthetic injection of the AC joint itself. See Chapter 8 for a description of these injection tests.

The vertical stability of the AC joint is then tested by alternately pushing up and pulling down on the arm while carefully palpating the joint with two fin-

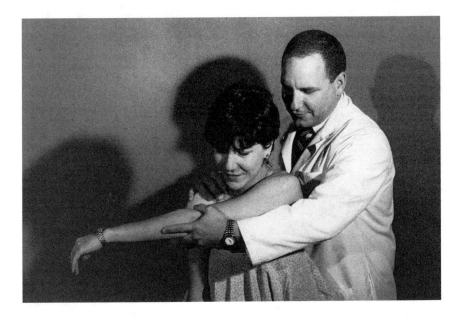

**Figure 2–6** Horizontal adduction test.

gers on the clavicle and two on the acromion (Figure 2–7). More than approximately 5 mm of motion is evidence of AC separation.

### GH Joint

The true ball-and-socket joint of the shoulder is bounded by confluent flat tendons behind and above (the rotator cuff tendons) and in front (the subscapularis tendon). The GH joint is most easily palpated from its posterior surface with the examiner's ipsilateral thumb. The GH joint line is palpated posteriorly in a soft spot that is found approximately 2 cm inferior and 2 cm medial to the posterolateral corner of the acromion (Figure 2–8). The posterolateral corner of the acromion is termed the acromial angle. It is the most reliable bony landmark around the shoulder in patients with thick subcutaneous fat around the shoulder, in whom palpation of any bony landmarks at all can be difficult. The acromial angle is palpated with the pads of the examiner's ipsilateral thumb and forefinger held together as if to pinch something (Figure

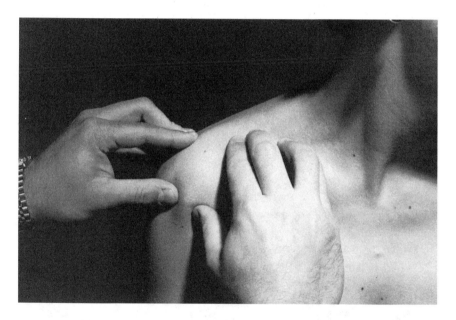

**Figure 2–7** Test of vertical stability of the AC joint. A fingertip directly on the superior aspect of the joint can detect subtle motion as the clavicle is alternately depressed and released.

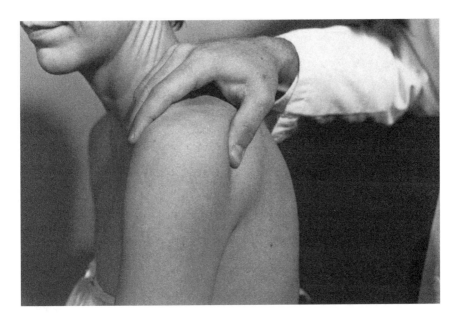

**Figure 2–8** Palpation for GH joint line tenderness.

2–9). These two fingers can feel the simultaneous pressure of the lateral and posterior surfaces of the acromion remarkably well, even if they are feeling through thick adipose tissue.

The acromial angle's relationship to the GH joint line is used by the surgeon when beginning arthroscopy to determine the point of entry into the posterior GH joint. This is the same point that is palpated in physical examination of the posterior joint line. Pain produced by pressure at this location is found with instability and any condition that produces irritation of the joint's lining tissue (the synovium). Infection, arthritis, and intraarticular bleeding are common causes. Posterior joint line tenderness is, along with loss of external rotation range, a classic sign of GH arthritis. In formal terminology, synovitis produces true posterior capsular tenderness, and instability produces the pain of subluxation. Both produce pain when pressure is applied to the posterior joint line, but pain of a different nature, the former being more of a soreness and the latter a sharp pain associated with the bad proprioceptive information that something is going "out of place."

The humeral shaft is next rotated by the examiner's ipsilateral on the patient's elbow. The contralateral hand is placed with the palm on the acromion, the thumb on the posterior joint line, and the fingers on the anterior

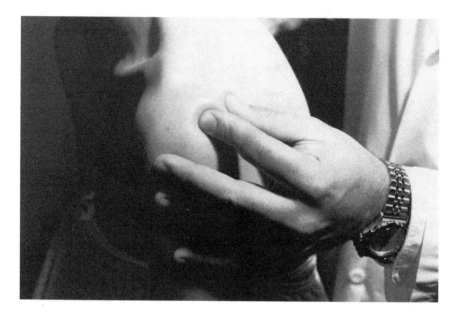

**Figure 2–9** Palpation for the posterior acromial angle. This is the most reliable bony landmark of the shoulder.

---

joint line (with the examiner still standing behind the seated patient). In this position, the roughness of the GH articulation and any catches, pops, or grinds can be best felt by the hand on the shoulder. Complete relaxation of the deltoid and cuff is essential for this examination to be sensitive. This is encouraged by strong, firm support of the patient's entire upper extremity by the examiner's ipsilateral hand. This GH grinding maneuver (Figure 2–10), performed in multiple positions of forward elevation and abduction-adduction, is one of the most sensitive tests for intraarticular loose bodies and labral tears.

By this point in the examination, the examiner is becoming oriented to the plane of the acromion and may start to visualize the course of the rotator cuff muscles and tendons as they originate on the scapula, course under the distal clavicle and acromion, and terminate on the greater tuberosity of the humerus. The plane of the acromion varies enormously among individuals; it is horizontal in some and nearly vertical in others. It must be appreciated, however, to examine for the common malady of subacromial impingement.

The bony architecture of the shoulder girdle can be nearly impossible to palpate in some fat and muscular patients. As mentioned, the most reliable landmark is the posterolateral corner of the acromion. It can be felt in nearly

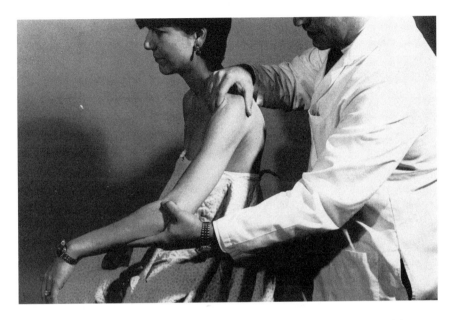

**Figure 2–10** GH grinding maneuver. Rotation and gentle compression of the joint are applied with one hand on the patient's arm. The examiner palpates with the other hand on the GH joint line.

everyone. From here the lateral edge and then the anterolateral corner of this flat bone are found. Tenderness along the margins of the acromion is sought. It is most important along the anterior edge because here, under the deltoid, is generally where the rotator cuff impinges against both the overhanging lip of the acromion and the coracoclavicular ligament, which arises from it. Acromial marginal tenderness is often, but not always, present in impingers. It is a dominant feature in patients with calcific rotator cuff tendinitis, generally of a much brighter (ie, painful) quality.

With the acromion well in hand, the impingement test[2] is now done by maintaining downward pressure on the forward edge of the acromion while lifting or elevating the arm to greater than 150° (Figure 2–11). Pain felt as the rotator cuff jams into the undersurface of the downpressed acromion represents a positive test result.

The greater tuberosity of the humerus is palpable anteriorly with the arm externally rotated at the patient's side. Just medial to this is the bicipital groove, containing the tendon of the long head of the biceps. This is tender, as one might guess, in cases of bicipital tendinitis. There is also significant ten-

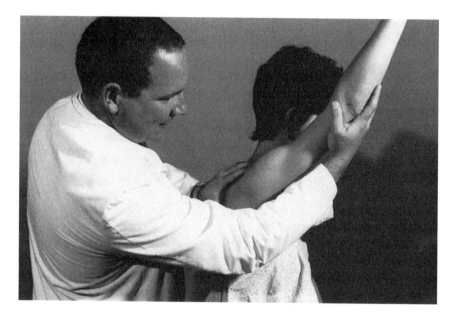

**Figure 2–11** Impingement test.

derness at nearly the same location after an acute anterior dislocation. True palpation of the biceps tendon may be possible in some thin people, but keep in mind that this tendon is about the diameter of a Cross pen and is protected by the bony tuberosities and the thick, multipenniform deltoid muscle. Bicipital tendon tenderness can be determined by repeated palpation of the area just below the tuberosities in internal and external rotation (do this in both rotations to keep from confusing anterior GH joint line tenderness from biceps tendon tenderness). The rolling, linear structure that is palpated in front of the shoulder is far more likely to be one of the segments of the anterior deltoid, however.

With the cumulative stereognostic information from the preceding parts of the examination, the examiner is prepared for the most subtle part: examination for stability of the GH joint. This is first done from behind the seated patient and is then repeated with the patient supine. Anterior stability is first evaluated by a maneuver termed shucking (Figure 2–12). The ipsilateral hand pushes the humeral head forward and backward while the contralateral hand stabilizes the entire scapula and provides the examiner the tactile feedback to know that he or she is actually translating the humeral head with respect to the glenoid and not merely pulling and pushing the entire scapula around on the thorax. The arm is then pulled straight down while the examiner feels the lat-

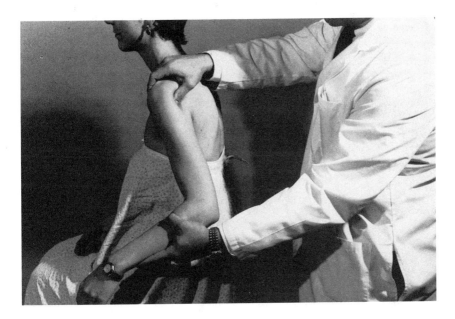

**Figure 2–12**  Anterior shucking or drawer maneuver.

eral edge of the acromion. Downward translation greater than that produced in the other shoulder and the appearance of an indentation below the edge of the acromion (the sulcus sign; Figure 2–13) are signs of inferior GH instability. Posterior instability is detected by the presence of pain with direct posterior pressure, with both a shucking maneuver and direct posterior pressure on the forward flexed arm.

Anterior instability, by far the most common type, also produces pain with forced external rotation of the arm when held at the side. This pain stops when direct posterior pressure is placed on the humeral head from the front (known as the relocation test). The classic sign of anterior instability, known as the apprehension sign, is the sudden tightening of the shoulder girdle muscles, accompanied by a grimace, when the abducted, externally rotated humerus is forcefully pushed forward. This should be done slowly to prevent true dislocation.

## SCAPULOTHORACIC ARTICULATION

The unclothed back of the shoulder patient should be observed carefully as the patient moves the shoulder through maximal active arcs of forward elevation, abduction, and internal and external rotation. Although modesty (and

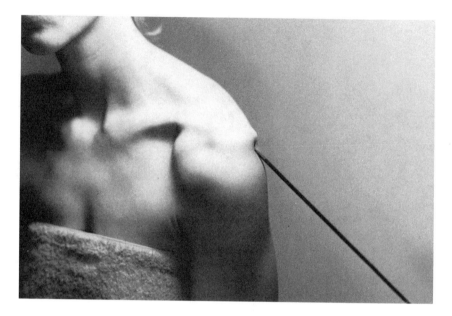

**Figure 2–13** Sulcus sign.

perhaps laziness) often argues against doing this, it is important that each person responsible for examining a patient do this at least once. Many of the common diagnoses can be made with the eyes alone. Winging of the scapula can usually be appreciated in the standing patient. It can be made more prominent by having the patient lean against a wall with the elbows locked in extension. Winging generally indicates dysfunction of the serratus anterior or its innervation, the long thoracic nerve. The scapula may be fixed in position by a congenital bony bar (termed Sprengel's deformity). Longstanding scapulothoracic bursitis often produces a lump at the lower angle. All are diagnoses made merely by observation.

The fullness of the scapular fossae, where the muscular bellies of the supraspinatus and infraspinatus muscles are located, is noted. The supraspinatus fossa, in particular, is commonly decreased in bulk in cases of longstanding rotator cuff tear. Symmetry of the spine and shoulder girdles is regarded; doing this regularly will teach the examiner the usual asymmetry that accompanies hand dominance in most athletes. Despite the great deal that is spoken about the scapulothoracic rhythm, there is no reproducibly good way of examining it. This term refers to the rotation of the scapula as a function of the position of the shoulder. It definitely can be seen to be different in painful shoulders than in nonpainful ones. It also changes with speed of elevation of the shoulder, the relative abduction of the shoulder during elevation, the athletic background of the patient, and the position of the patient's neck during elevation. Paralysis of the muscles that move the scapula, trauma, and rotator cuff disease also affect it. The only finding that seems to have reproducible value on the general physical examination of the shoulder is therefore increased or decreased scapular movement on shoulder abduction relative to the unaffected side.

Careful palpation is the most important part of the scapulothoracic examination. Palpate first lightly for spasm and then more deeply for masses and tenderness. Feel for crepitus as the scapula is actively moved about the back. With the arms maximally adducted, the area that is normally between the scapula and the chest wall is exposed. This is where scapulothoracic bursitis is most tender. The scapulothoracic syndrome of Michele[3] is indicated by tenderness at this point. The rhomboids insert near this area, and there is often a tender lump, palpable near the scapula's medial inferior border, that is most assuredly not bursal tissue. Cervical nerve root compression often produces pain and spasm of the small muscles in this area. On the other edge of the scapula, the origin of the triceps may be tender locally. The tubercle of Lushka[4] is a bony prominence, often tender to palpation, on the superomedial border of the scapula. A benign bony growth called an osteochondroma may grow anywhere on the scapula and is often palpable.

The true, scientific evidence for most of the periscapular pain syndromes being caused by the entities described is in fact quite tenuous. Nonetheless, by always asking "Is this like your pain?" as tender, lumpy areas are found, the careful examiner of the scapulothoracic area will produce grateful patients. Although poorly (if at all) understood, these tender lumps respond well to specifically directed physical treatments.

## MUSCLE TESTING

Range of motion testing, which is probably the single most important element of the shoulder examination, is included under muscle testing because both passive and active motion is routinely tested. Muscular resistance often influences the recorded passive range end points as well. Range of motion should be tested at every examination. The passive range is recorded first. Forward elevation in neutral rotation and external rotation with the arm at the side are recorded in degrees. Internal rotation is recorded as how far up the spine (to which spinal level) the patient can raise his or her thumbnail. These basic three data are recorded in shorthand (eg, RA170/65/t8 meaning "right shoulder active range of motion: forward elevation, 170°; external rotation,

65°; internal rotation, thumbnail to eighth thoracic level"). Other ranges may be recorded in specific instances, such as extension, abduction, and adduction ranges. It is remarkable how infrequently these other data are of any real clinical consequence, however.

Two subtleties enter into the range of motion test. The first is maintaining an awareness for scapular and spine motion that helps elevate the arm. Many shoulder patients, involved in a program to increase range progressively, will attempt to please the practitioner (and get themselves out of some painful stretching) by protracting the scapula and extending the lumbar spine to get their perceived forward elevation range up. Although few people have the ability to isolate GH motion like a ballerina, the normal amount of compensatory motion in raising the arm may be recognized by experience and looking at the other side. Excessive spine or scapular motion should be noted and an estimate of the true forward elevation made.

The other subtlety in range testing is recognition of the end point (ie, how hard one should push). It is most important to push with the same firmness in each examination on a given patient and to relax the patient and push with a firmness appropriate to habitus and pain. This may be illustrated by the fact that a fairly vigorous push to end point is needed to record range of motion in a 400-pound bench press champion and that a rather gentler touch is used on a rheumatoid patient 2 weeks after total shoulder surgery.

The strength and coordinate control of the shoulder girdle muscles under resistive feedback testing are essential elements of the diagnostic examination. Isometric resistive feedback, meaning that the patient applies more and more force as the examiner pushes back harder, is more rapid, possibly less harmful, and more likely to reflect accurately the strength of the muscle or group being tested than graduated isotonic or most isokinetic testing methods. Although the isokinetic apparatus has a place in training, its need in the routine examination and rehabilitation of shoulders is limited.

The most important muscles on which to have strength data recorded in the physical examination are the trapezius/levator scapulae, deltoid (three parts), rotator cuff group (two parts), subscapularis, and biceps brachii. Strength of the scapular rotators is difficult to test and not very reproducible. Here, the absence of winging and symmetric scapular motion are the most commonly needed elements of the muscle examination. The trapezius group is tested by pushing down on the acromia as the patient attempts to shrug the shoulders up. A standard five-level scale is satisfactory (1, trace or palpable contraction without movement; 2, movement but insufficient to overcome gravity; 3, just able to overcome gravity; 4, overcoming gravity but abnormally weak; 5, within normal limits; + and – as appropriate). The anterior, middle, and posterior deltoids are tested with the elbow flexed, with the arm at the side, and by feedback resistive flexion, abduction, and extension of the shoulder. The patient's ability to set the scapula obviously will affect this test. In the rare case that the scapula cannot be set (ie, held immobile on the chest to permit a firm base for testing the deltoid), the patient may be placed supine with a pad of folded towels under the ipsilateral scapula to immobilize it.

The rotator cuff is herein considered to consist of three confluent tendons: the supraspinatus, infraspinatus, and teres minor. The subscapularis tendon, although listed as part of the rotator cuff in most texts, is in so many ways a different structure that it is always referred to separately and by name in this book. The rotator cuff is tested first by a supraspinatus isolation maneuver (Figure 2–14). The elbow is held in extension, and the arm is internally rotated maximally and forward elevated about 70° (forward elevation is raising the arm in the plane of the scapula, that is, anatomic flexion in approximately 30° of abduction). Care should be taken to rotate internally maximally. This neutralizes the ability of the deltoid to contribute to the elevation. Merely asking the patient to point the thumb to the floor is insufficient to do this. This supraspinatus isolation is a test of the anterior cuff. The posterior cuff is tested by the patient resisting external rotation, starting at neutral, with the arm at the side. The subscapularis is then tested (Figure 2–15) by asking the patient to

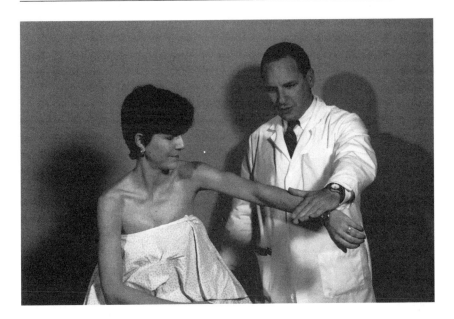

**Figure 2–14** Supraspinatus isolation maneuver.

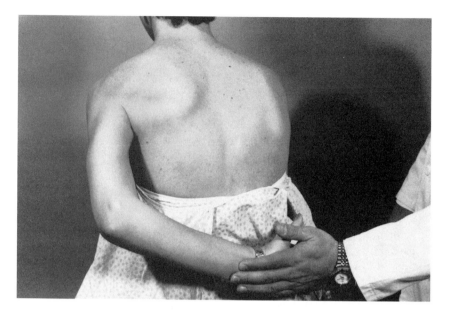

**Figure 2–15** Subscapularis isolation maneuver.

lift the dorsum of the hand off the midlumbar back. Because there are so many (neutralized) powerful internal rotators of the humerus, and because this position is so near the maximum range of GH internal rotation, normal strength may be a surprisingly small amount of force.

The commonly quoted "painful arc" sign of rotator cuff tear is an unreliable sign on which to base this diagnosis. The report of pain through a specific range of the abduction arc in active abduction of the shoulder was thought to indicate rotator cuff tear because these muscles were thought to be inactive at the initiation and termination of the abduction arc. Although it may commonly be observed, this sign is not routinely sought because so many conditions other than rotator cuff tear may produce it and because so many patients with cuff tears do not display it. Experience will teach the thoughtful examiner to recognize quickly the patient with rotator cuff pain. There are many ways of compensating for a deficient cuff to achieve functional movements using the deltoid and scapular rotators. The classic appearance of the patient with complete disruption of the rotator cuff—hiking up the entire shoulder girdle and bending at the trunk just to get the arm up to shake hands—is not very common. Most patients with a large cuff tear compensate fairly well. Indeed, part of the nonoperative treatment of rotator cuff tear involves enhancing this compensatory use of the other shoulder girdle muscles. It is safe practice to avoid ranging, strengthening, and even most testing in anatomic abduction. Abduction maximizes shoulder joint reaction forces, anterior dislocation forces, subacromial impingement force, and stretch of the capsule.

The biceps brachii is tested regularly because its long head is such an efficient depressor of the humeral head (humeral head depression decreases subacromial impingement of the rotator cuff). Palpate the muscle belly of the biceps, and observe for symmetry to check for rupture of the proximal tendon, which occurs frequently in impingers. Stabilize the arm against extension with the contralateral hand (stand in front of the patient), and have the patient flex the elbow against resistance given by the ipsilateral hand. The ipsilateral hand may then be used to grip the patient's hand as in a handshake, and the patient is asked to supinate the pronated forearm forcefully. This also tests the biceps, which is a powerful supinator as well as flexor of the elbow. In cases of biceps tendinitis, both these maneuvers will be accompanied by pain. This opens the last segment of the shoulder examination, which is termed provocative testing or resisted isolated muscle testing and is done to evaluate pain caused by contraction.

Inflammation or tearing anywhere within the musculotendinous unit tends to produce pain on resisted contraction of that unit. Each muscle tested in the shoulder examination may therefore be subjected to provocative testing by noting pain during contraction. Also important is the sense of how much or what fraction of maximal contraction is needed to produce the pain and how closely the pain thus produced resembles the patient's typical pain. Of special importance in this area is the rotator cuff. The supraspinatus isolation maneuver (see above) may produce pain after nearly any acute shoulder trauma. This may be due to trauma to the cuff itself, the fact that the cuff muscles cause large joint reaction forces when isometrically contracting, or twisting of the deltoid in this position. Regardless of the cause, after X-rays have ruled out fracture, provocative testing of the cuff in any acutely painful shoulder should be done in multiple positions of elevation, abduction, and rotation.

If forced external rotation in multiple positions is painful and the pain is of the same quality, it is likely to be related to acute cuff injury. More chronic cuff pathology tends to produce a constant level of pain with provocative testing of the isolated supraspinatus. The pain is often felt at the deltoid insertion area in the upper third of the arm. Deltoid tendinitis produces pain in this area with resisted arm flexion or abduction from neutral position. More significant, there is tenderness at the deltoid insertion, something that is never found with cuff pain referred to the deltoid insertion. Generally, the combination of tenderness and pain with resisted contraction indicates muscle injury. Many other specific overuse syndromes about the shoulder can be logically diagnosed with these data from provocative testing.

## INJECTION TESTING

Although diagnosis of shoulder pain is often much more difficult than pain in the other major joints, injection testing does offer a way to test one's diagnostic hypotheses. Three major areas of injection testing about the shoulder are frequently employed: the subacromial, GH, and AC injections. Occasionally, injection of the biceps tendon in the intertubercular sulcus of the humerus is performed, but this is primarily a therapeutic injection for the already established diagnosis of bicipital tendinitis. Although these injection tests are usually performed by physicians, the results of the tests should always be known by the treating therapist. Injection testing generally provides the most reliable diagnostic information available.

Injection testing relies on the use of a local anesthetic solution (usually 1% lidocaine) delivered to a specific, known location. If the patient's symptoms are relieved by the injection or if a specific painful maneuver is rendered painless by the injection, the injection test is said to be positive. Any injection test may be performed with the addition of a steroid compound to the solution for a local antiinflammatory effect. More is mentioned regarding this in Chapter 5.

The most commonly performed injection test is that of the subacromial space. A positive subacromial injection test is a reliable indicator of the impingement diagnosis. First, an impingement test is performed as described above. The posterior aspect of the shoulder is then prepared for injection with alcohol or povidone iodine solution, and approximately 7 mL of local anesthetic is injected into the space between the acromion and the rotator cuff (Figure 2–16). The needle is withdrawn, and about a minute later the impingement test is repeated. If the patient no longer experiences pain with the impingement maneuver, the test is termed positive, and the diagnosis of subacromial impingement is made. The strength of the rotator cuff is also measured before and after the injection. Improvement in cuff strength after the injection indicates that rotator cuff pain is a limiting factor in the testing of its strength and that at least some of the cuff must be intact. Rotator cuff strength does not improve after subacromial injection in cases of large, longstanding tears or avulsion injuries involving the entire rotator cuff.

GH joint injection testing (Figure 2–17) involves injection of a similar amount of anesthetic into the GH joint cavity. This is done in suspected cases of pain from labral tearing or mild GH arthritis. Improvement in symptoms, as before, indicates a positive test, and the diagnosis of pain related to intra-

derness and pain with resisted contraction indicates muscle injury. Many other specific overuse syndromes about the shoulder can be logically diagnosed with these data from provocative testing.

## INJECTION TESTING

Although diagnosis of shoulder pain is often much more difficult than pain in the other major joints, injection testing does offer a way to test one's diagnostic hypotheses. Three major areas of injection testing about the shoulder are frequently employed: the subacromial, GH, and AC injections. Occasionally, injection of the biceps tendon in the intertubercular sulcus of the humerus is performed, but this is primarily a therapeutic injection for the already established diagnosis of bicipital tendinitis. Although these injection tests are usually performed by physicians, the results of the tests should always be known by the treating therapist. Injection testing generally provides the most reliable diagnostic information available.

Injection testing relies on the use of a local anesthetic solution (usually 1% lidocaine) delivered to a specific, known location. If the patient's symptoms are relieved by the injection or if a specific painful maneuver is rendered painless by the injection, the injection test is said to be positive. Any injection test may be performed with the addition of a steroid compound to the solution for a local antiinflammatory effect. More is mentioned regarding this in Chapter 5.

The most commonly performed injection test is that of the subacromial space. A positive subacromial injection test is a reliable indicator of the impingement diagnosis. First, an impingement test is performed as described above. The posterior aspect of the shoulder is then prepared for injection with alcohol or povidone iodine solution, and approximately 7 mL of local anesthetic is injected into the space between the acromion and the rotator cuff (Figure 2–16). The needle is withdrawn, and about a minute later the impingement test is repeated. If the patient no longer experiences pain with the impingement maneuver, the test is termed positive, and the diagnosis of subacromial impingement is made. The strength of the rotator cuff is also measured before and after the injection. Improvement in cuff strength after the injection indicates that rotator cuff pain is a limiting factor in the testing of its strength and that at least some of the cuff must be intact. Rotator cuff strength does not improve after subacromial injection in cases of large, longstanding tears or avulsion injuries involving the entire rotator cuff.

GH joint injection testing (Figure 2–17) involves injection of a similar amount of anesthetic into the GH joint cavity. This is done in suspected cases of pain from labral tearing or mild GH arthritis. Improvement in symptoms, as before, indicates a positive test, and the diagnosis of pain related to intra-

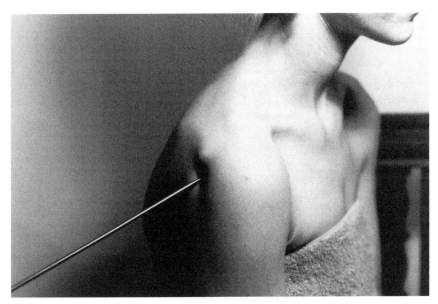

**Figure 2–16** Subacromial injection. The pointer indicates the placement and direction of the needle.

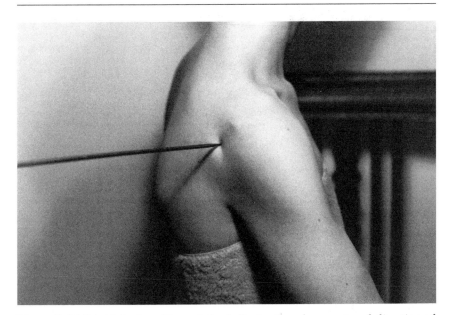

**Figure 2–17** Joint injection. The pointer indicates the placement and direction of the needle.

articular pathology may be made. It is good practice, however, to perform a subacromial injection first to see which of the patient's symptoms and/or clinical signs are relieved. If there is a significant full-thickness tear of the rotator cuff, fluid injected into the GH joint will flow through the tear into the subacromial space, confusing the issue of whether the patient's pain is being generated here or in the GH joint. The information from the subacromial injection will prevent this confusion.

As noted earlier, impingement itself may produce some pain with horizontal adduction or grind, causing confusion with the pain of AC arthritis. The horizontal adduction test should therefore be done before and after any subacromial injection to see if the AC joint really is the source of pain. If, after subacromial injection, the AC joint is still tender and pain is still produced with horizontal adduction, the AC joint injection test (Figure 2–18) can be used to verify the diagnosis of AC arthritic pain. In this test, the same local anesthetic, usually with some added steroid, is injected directly into the AC joint cavity. A much smaller volume is used here. If horizontal adduction no longer produces pain, the test is termed positive, and the diagnosis of AC arthritis is verified.

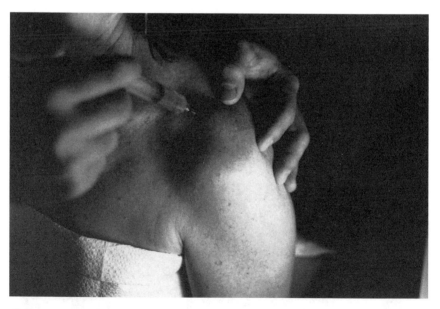

**Figure 2–18** AC joint injection.

**REFERENCES**

1. Robbins SL, Angell M, Vinas K. *Basic Pathology*. Philadelphia, Pa: Saunders; 1981.
2. Neer CS II. Anterior acromioplasty for the chronic impingement syndrome in the shoulder. *J Bone Joint Surg Am*. 1972;54:41–49.
3. Michele AA, Davis JJ, Krueger FJ, Lientor JM. Scapulocostal syndrome. *N-Y J Med*. 1950;50:1353–1357.
4. Butters KP. The scapula. In: Rockwood CA, Matsen FA, eds. *The Shoulder*. Philadelphia, Pa: Saunders; 1990:363.

# Chapter 3

# Radiographic Examination of the Shoulder

## PLAIN FILMS

Regular X-rays are routinely taken in hospital emergency departments and orthopaedic offices. They provide much specific information about the calcified tissues about the shoulder, most notably the bones. Fractures, dislocations, and most cases of arthritis can be diagnosed by plain films alone. Soft tissue problems about the shoulder are much more common, however, and here the information from plain films is mostly inferential; that is, signs seen on X-rays are consistent with, but not diagnostic of, the ligamentous and musculotendinous problems encountered about the shoulder.

Most shoulder fractures are readily diagnosed by plain films. There is some advantage to performing a perfunctory examination of the shoulder before radiographic evaluation, however. Reproducible bony tenderness after trauma is probably caused by fracture. Even the often-reported "bone bruise" is usually a small, localized, traumatic disruption of the bone's normal architecture (ie, a fracture). Periosteum, the membrane that covers bone, is richly innervated about the shoulder. Much of the pain of a fracture comes from irritation of the local periosteum. The physical finding of reproducible bony tenderness at the greater tuberosity often prompts a careful reexamination of X-rays, initially read as negative for fracture, with the finding of a non-displaced (ie, fragments not separated) fracture of the greater tuberosity then being noted (Figure 3–1).

Although it is not common for practitioners other than orthopaedists and radiologists to refer to films, physical findings of other physicians and therapists that are not consistent with a reported diagnosis should prompt a focused review of all the available diagnostic information, including X-rays in any traumatic case demonstrating true bony tenderness.

Many X-ray views of the shoulder are obtained by shoulder surgeons for special purposes of evaluating specific small bony deformities and clearances.

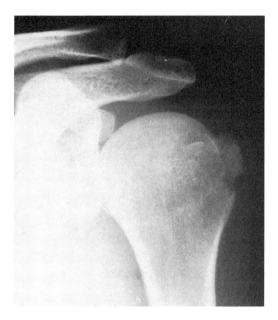

**Figure 3–1** Radiograph showing a nondisplaced fracture of the greater tuberosity of the humerus. This fracture was unseen on a standard rotational view.

There are three standard views with which all members of the health care team ought to be familiar, and from which the vast majority of X-ray diagnoses can be made: anteroposterior (AP), lateral, and axillary (Figures 3–2 through 3–4). The most important of these is the AP view. The AP shoulder film shows the shoulder girdle as it would be seen if one were facing the patient. Most fractures and dislocations show up on this view, as do calcific changes in the rotator cuff tendons (Figure 3–5). The relative thickness of the acromion can be seen along with changes on its undersurface that might cause impingement on the rotator cuff (Figure 3–6). Arthritic changes of the acromioclavicular joint (Figure 3–7) and the glenohumeral joint (Figure 3–8) as well as irregularities of the clavicle that would result from an old fracture or a tumor are usually visible on this view.

AP views of the shoulder can be made with the humerus in different degrees of internal and external rotation to demonstrate irregularities of the humeral head, such as the Hill-Sachs deformity (Figure 3–9). This is a denting of the posterior aspect of the humeral head that is produced by the anterior aspect of the glenoid when the humeral head is dislocated anteriorly. More is said about this in Chapter 9.

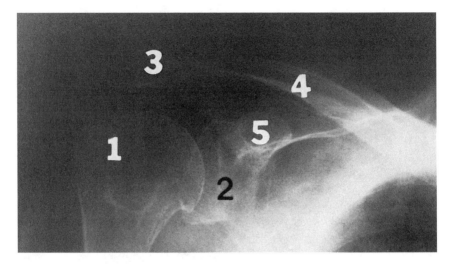

**Figure 3–2** Normal radiographic AP projection. 1, humeral head; 2, glenoid; 3, acromion; 4, clavicle; 5, coracoid process.

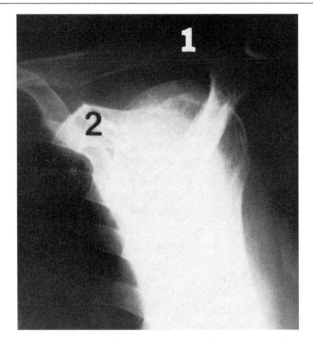

**Figure 3–3** Normal radiographic lateral projection. 1, acromion; 2, coracoid process.

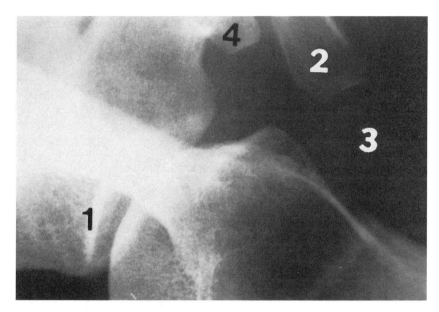

**Figure 3–4** Normal radiographic axillary projection. 1, glenoid; 2, clavicle; 3, acromion; 4, coracoid process.

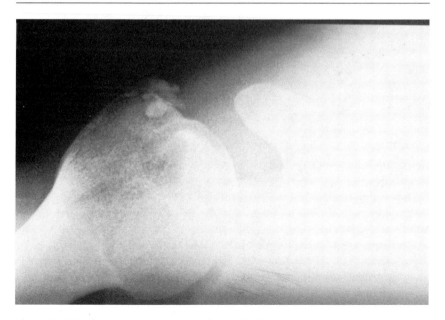

**Figure 3–5** Radiograph showing calcific tendinitis.

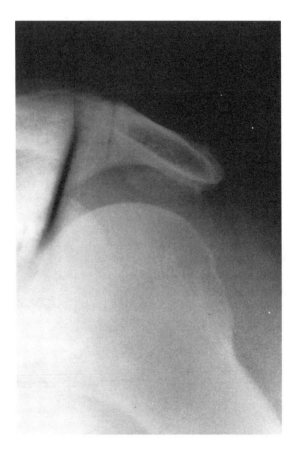

**Figure 3–6** Radiograph showing bony projections (spurs) on the inferior surface of the acromion, which produce impingement on the underlying rotator cuff.

The lateral view of the scapula, or the scapular Y view, shows the flat scapula on edge (see Figure 3–3). This is an easy film to take, and it can pick up fractures of the scapular processes (the acromion, coracoid, and glenoid) that other views miss. It will also demonstrate the direction of dislocation of the humeral head relative to the glenoid.

The third view that is important to diagnosis is the axillary view (see Figure 3–4). Although this is not a standard view in many radiology departments, it ought to be because no other view demonstrates the glenohumeral relationship as plainly. The axillary also picks up anterior and posterior glenoid rim fractures that would otherwise be missed by plain films.

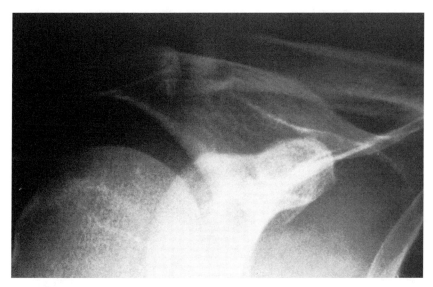

**Figure 3–7** Radiograph showing acromioclavicular arthritis.

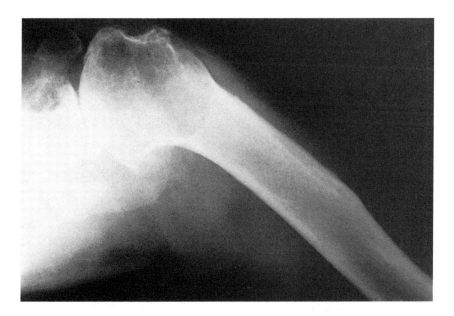

**Figure 3–8** Radiograph showing glenohumeral osteoarthritis.

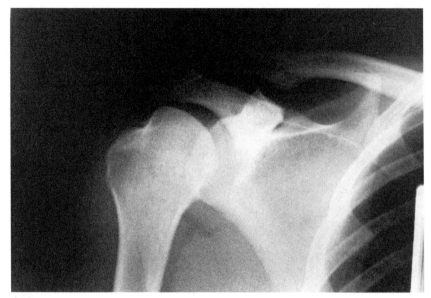

A

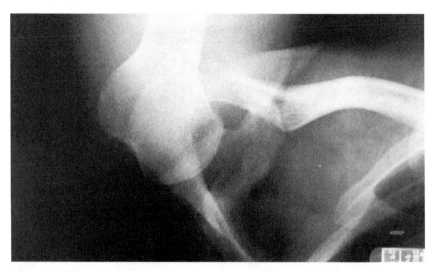

B

**Figure 3–9  (A)** Anteroposterior radiograph showing Hill-Sachs lesion, an indentation of the humeral head produced by the anterior glenoid during anterior dislocation. **(B)** Axillary view radiograph showing same lesion.

A particularly important reason for obtaining plain films of the shoulder in the nontraumatic setting is for the demonstration of the calcific deposits associated with acute calcific tendinitis (see Figure 3–5). This is a reasonably common cause of acute, severe pain that is associated with a specific point of extreme tenderness on physical examination. Multiple rotational AP views are obtained if this is suspected to help localize the calcific deposits.

Postfracture follow-up and postoperative X-rays after any bony reconstructive procedure, such as open reduction with internal fixation or joint replacement, are important to the therapists involved in the patient's rehabilitation. The aggressiveness with which increased range of motion may be pursued can be judged by the degree of healing seen on plain film. Knowledge that what has been done so far has not disrupted a bony construct is itself quite helpful. Healing of fractures is estimated on plain films by the presence of callus, the calcified repair tissue of bone. The typical X-ray appearance of this is seen in Figure 3–10. Tissue that is essentially callus may form de novo in muscular or capsular tissues, especially after trauma. This phenomenon, termed heterotopic ossification, is often present in patients with posttraumatic loss of shoulder motion. It is especially common if there has been severe head injury. These chunks of bone may be responsible for blocking motion in some cases. The plain film is an excellent way to follow the progress of therapies used for heterotopic bone. The other radiologic tool of use here is the radionuclide bone scan.

## RADIONUCLIDE BONE SCAN

The living cells of bone that are responsible for producing the calcified bony matrix that is visible on plain film X-rays are called osteoblasts. They obviously must utilize calcium. Molecules that the osteoblast treats as calcium may be tagged with radioactive atoms, whose location can then be determined with a sensor of the radioactivity produced by these atoms. This is the principle behind bone scanning. In practice, the bone scan is "hot" anywhere bone is in a state of increased metabolism. This means anywhere there is a fracture, arthritis, infection, or active bone growth, such as sites of heterotopic ossification or simply growing bone in a child. Cancer patients are frequently scanned to check for the presence of bone metastases. In patients suspected of having a fracture but in whom plain films fail to demonstrate a clear-cut fracture, the bone scan being "cold" can definitely rule out a fracture. A scan that is "hot" at the point of bony tenderness (Figure 3–11) usually confirms the diagnosis of fracture. The bone scans generally in use expose patients to little more radiation than they would receive in a chest X-ray. Although certainly not considered routine studies, they are in common use and provide reliable information

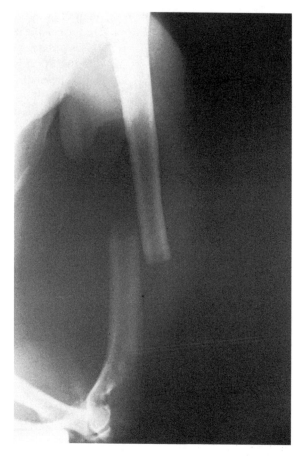

A

**Figure 3–10 (A)** Radiograph showing early fracture healing with callus formation.

---

in questions about tumor (Figure 3–12) and occult fracture. It should be kept in mind that acromioclavicular joints in older patients routinely have a "hot" appearance on bone scan that rarely corresponds to symptomatic acromioclavicular arthritis.

## ARTHROGRAMS

For years, the arthrogram of the shoulder was a standard test used to determine the presence of rotator cuff tear (Figure 3–13). In this test, the

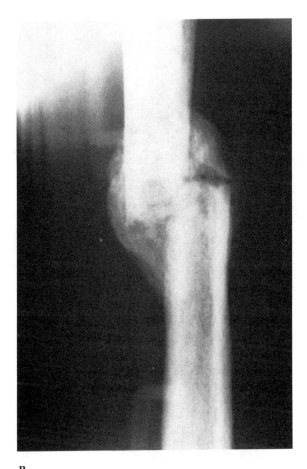

**B**

**Figure 3–10 (B)** Radiograph showing late fracture healing with callus formation.

---

glenohumeral joint is injected with a radiopaque (ie, visible on plain film X-ray) dye. Plain films are then taken, and if the dye has leaked out of the glenohumeral joint the assumption is made that there must be a hole in the rotator cuff (and capsule) that is permitting the leak (Figure 3–14). This is an accurate, specific, but limited test. It answers the question of whether a rotator cuff tear exists. In modern practice it has been supplanted by magnetic resonance (MR) imaging because of the greater amount of information this gives. There is also no injection and no risk of allergy to the iodine-containing dye.

Arthrograms do not give reliable information about the size of rotator cuff tears, nor do they tell much more than plain films about the other soft tissue

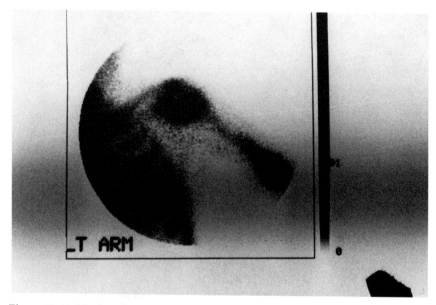

**Figure 3–11** Nuclear bone scan using $^{99m}$Tc showing a fracture of the humeral shaft, indicated by increased local pick-up of isotope.

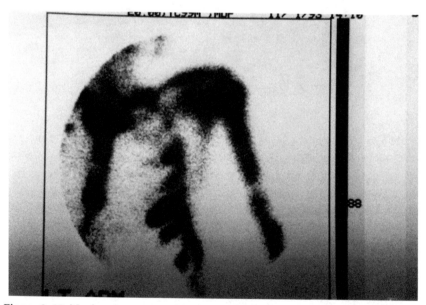

**Figure 3–12** Nuclear bone scan showing multiple metastases to bone. These appear as "hot spots" on the scan.

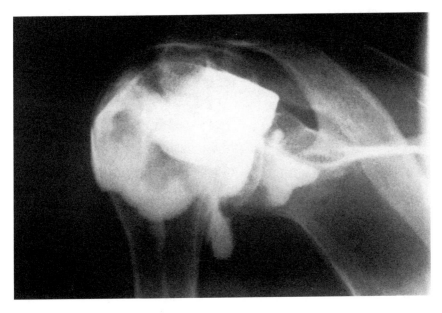

**Figure 3–13** Normal arthrogram.

structures in the shoulder. They are the test of choice for certain cystic (hollow) tumors around the shoulder or for patients with rotator cuff signs who cannot stand to be confined in an MR machine. They are also much cheaper than MR scans.

The computed tomography (CT) arthrogram is made by performing CT scans of the shoulder after injecting dye as for a normal arthrogram. This is the most sensitive test for tearing of the glenoid labrum, although it, too, is being supplanted by MR scanning as the latter is technologically improved.

## MR AND CT SCANS

CT provides horizontal (ie, parallel to the floor if one were examining a standing patient) slice pictures of the shoulder that have excellent bony definition (better, in fact, than MR scans) but rather poor soft tissue definition (Figure 3–15). They are obtained in cases of glenoid fracture and scapular fracture and use an injected contrast (as for the arthrogram) to visualize the glenoid labrum. Quite a lot of radiation exposure is involved in CT scanning, and its routine use for shoulder patients is limited. The CT scan utilizes X-rays to create images, just as plain radiographs do. A completely different physical mechanism is used in the creation of MR images.

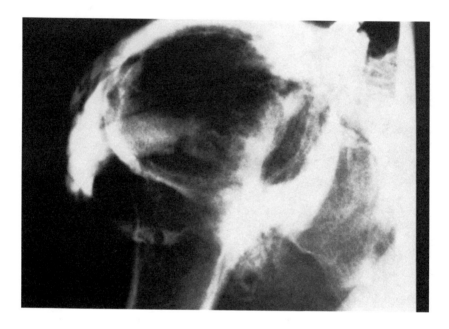

**Figure 3–14** Arthrogram showing a rotator cuff tear. Radiopaque dye present in the subacromial space or lateral to the greater tuberosity indicates extravasation from the glenohumeral joint via a torn rotator cuff and capsule.

MR imaging is being used with ever increasing frequency in nearly all branches of medicine. The shoulder is no exception. This technique uses a high-strength magnetic field and radio waves to produce images of tissues based on the relative density and chemical microenvironment of the hydrogen atoms they contain. Images can be produced in any plane. The rotator cuff can be imaged. Swelling and inflammation are noticeable in muscle, bone, and even tendon. MR imaging itself provides a tremendous amount of information. MR scan interpretation is another problem area, however.

Most MR scanners have attached to themselves radiologists, who are trained in the interpretation of radiographs. Because the majority of radiologists in practice finished their training before MR imaging was invented, their level of expertise in MR scan interpretation varies considerably. It is not unusual for two radiologists reading the same MR image to note different findings. The shoulder surgeon, who has a great deal of experience looking at MR films and then looking directly at the tissues at surgery, is also responsible for interpretation of these images. His or her interpretation may be more accurate than a given radiologist's.

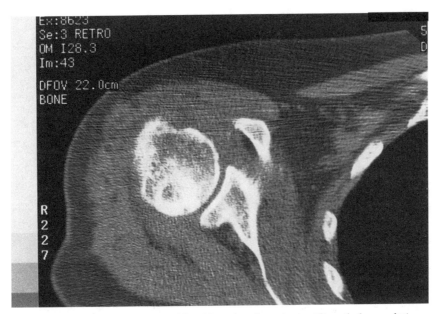

**Figure 3–15** CT scan of the shoulder. Note that there is significantly less soft tissue detail than that obtained by MR imaging.

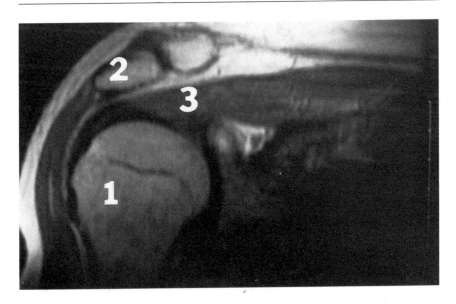

**Figure 3–16** Normal MR scan of the shoulder. 1, humeral head; 2, acromion; 3, rotator cuff.

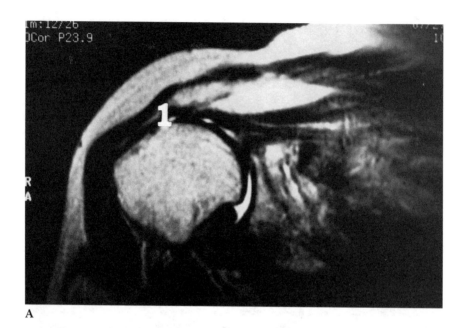

A

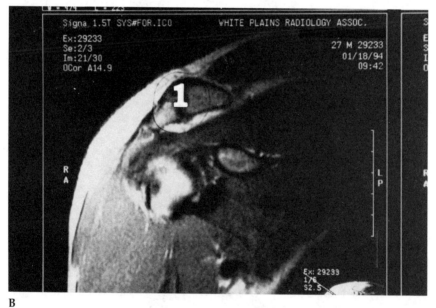

B

**Figure 3–17** MR scan of the shoulder. **(A)** Rotator cuff tear (1) indicated by lack of cuff signal. **(B)** Acromioclavicular joint arthritis (1) indicated by enlargement and inhomogeneous signal of the joint.

What is important here, however, is not who is better at MR scan interpretation but that the MR scan should generally be used as a confirmatory test for a diagnosis made by history, physical examination, and injection testing. Although there are certain pathologic entities seen on MR images that are not expected, such as occult tumors, these are rare. As mentioned earlier, MR readings may include findings that are not producing the patient's symptoms. They should therefore always be interpreted in light of physical findings.

It is unlikely that the practice of shoulder therapeutics would change dramatically if the MR image became completely unavailable. Nonetheless, the test is readily available at present and does provide a great wealth of information. This can create a greater level of confidence and comfort in the patient and all practitioners involved. For examples of typical MR image pathoanatomic findings, see Figures 3–16 and 3–17.

# Chapter 4

# Nonmusculoskeletal Causes of Shoulder Pain

## CARDIAC

It is of extreme importance that pain produced by cardiovascular insufficiency not be confused with musculoskeletal or neurologic pain felt about the shoulder. Angina or anginal equivalent pain commonly is felt in the left arm and occasionally in the right arm. It can be felt only in the forearm, neck, or jaw. Quite a few patients with angina say that they feel it in their shoulder. This pain is not associated with tenderness.[1] It does not change with position of the shoulder, arm, or neck. The pain usually decreases with the administration of rapidly acting nitrates, such as sublingual nitroglycerin (which the patient may very well be carrying in a pocket). Anginal equivalent shoulder pain is also commonly associated with vaguely abnormal feelings, flutterings, or palpations in the chest. The patient should be asked about this.

Any suspicion that a shoulder pain is heart related should prompt immediate medical attention. Even if a patient assures the therapist that he or she gets anginal pain commonly and is not particularly worried, no therapy of any type should be done until a new cardiac clearance is obtained. Ischemic and dysrhythmic cardiac diseases are common and may present in patients already under treatment for an established shoulder problem. A low threshold for obtaining cardiac evaluation is essential to safe practice.

Although heart problems can produce shoulder pain, it is distinctly unusual for shoulder problems to produce chest symptoms. Chest wall problems, such as rib fractures, inflammation of the costal (rib) cartilages, pectoralis muscle tears, or sprains produce local pain, but it is nearly always accompanied by tenderness. As above, any patient suspected of having cardiac pain should obviously receive emergency medical evaluation to rule out a cardiac source before any further shoulder work is done. Chest wall tenderness is one reassuring sign that the pain is not cardiac, however.

## ABDOMINAL

Irritation of the diaphragm produces pain in the ipsilateral shoulder. This pain may be related to respiratory movements (ie, it may be pleuritic). It does not change with shoulder motion. The pain is typically vaguely localized somewhere in the posterior shoulder area or under the scapula. It is of a deep nature and is described as a sharp ache similar in some respects to a cramp. There is often some upper abdominal tenderness present, and deep palpation of the abdomen may intensify the shoulder area pain. This type of diaphragmatic irritation may be caused by an abscess, hematoma, pleural effusion (fluid in the pleural space between the lung and the chest wall), or basilar pneumonia (infection of the lowermost segments of the lung). Gallbladder pathology, an ulcer on the posterior wall of the stomach, or pancreatic inflammation may also produce this type of referred shoulder pain. Dilatation of the transverse colon by bowel gas may produce severe pains felt in the chest (which are often mistaken for cardiac pain). These gas pains are commonly felt in the area around the shoulder, although their sudden, spasmodic nature and the rapidity with which they disappear make them unlikely to be mistaken for musculoskeletal shoulder pain.

## NEUROLOGIC

The shoulder often produces neck pain, and the neck often produces shoulder pain. This is one of the most frequent diagnostic traps for practitioners. Cervical nerve root irritation by disc material or bone usually gives neck pain in addition to pain felt along the course of the nerve. The neck pain may be slight, however, and there are patients in whom there is no pain as long as the neck is not moved excessively. It is unfortunately true that the patient is rare whose cervical radiculopathy produces a pure dermatomal pattern of referral.

The key to avoiding this confusion is the physical examination of the neck. Neck motion will increase the shoulder pain if it is truly neurologic in origin; it may increase the neck pain felt in subacromial cervicalgia (neck pain caused by intrinsic shoulder impingement pathology; see Chapter 8), but if the problem really is intrinsic to the shoulder, the shoulder pain will not be worsened by neck motion.

Pain and palpable spasm of the trapezius are quite nonspecific; they can accompany both shoulder impingement and cervical radiculopathy. Trapezius symptoms are commonly severe and may be the presenting complaint.[2] They also occur frequently on their own with no discernible neck or shoulder signs. The shoulder pain that many cervical radiculopathy patients have often turns out to be felt in the trapezius area on careful questioning. There is nonetheless a typical presentation of fourth and fifth root compression that consists of deep pain felt in the deltoid and humeral head area. These patients may grab the fleshy part of the upper arm and say "I feel it here" in exactly the same manner as rotator cuff patients. The impingement sign will be negative, however (unless there is concomitant subacromial impingement), and as mentioned above the pain will be intensified by pushing the neck to the ends of its range. Increased pain with axial compression has not been a reliable sign in these patients.

The coexistence of cervical radiculopathy and intrinsic shoulder pathology producing both types of pain is not particularly rare, nor is it difficult to recognize if the physical examination is done carefully. Injection tests are also valuable in these situations. It has long been noticed that proximal nerve compression in a limb tends to render other pathologic phenomena more painful in that limb. Thus the pain of some mild impingement, lateral epicondylitis, or wrist tendinitis tends to be more significant when there is a chronic nerve root irritation above them. Many patients say "This is my bad arm" (or leg) and may have had multiple surgical procedures or injections for well-defined and properly diagnosed problems up and down that limb. It is conjectured that the double crush phenomenon is to blame for this, in which proximal compression renders a nerve more susceptible to damage from distal compression. Yet the exaggerated symptoms from the distal pathologic entities in the limb need not be associated with nerve compression. Although its mechanism remains unclear, this phenomenon may be responsible for the high incidence of simultaneous intrinsic neck and shoulder symptoms.

Shingles (herpes zoster) is a viral disease caused by the same virus as chickenpox that produces pain in a dermatomal pattern along with vesicular (small, blisterlike) skin lesions in the same pattern. The skin lesions are often tiny or may be already healed when the patient presents, and the pain may be felt deep within the shoulder. It may be quite severe, but it is typically a neurogenic pain that does not change much with position or use of the muscles around the shoulder. Looking carefully for skin lesions in a roughly dermatomal pattern is the way to make this diagnosis.


## VASCULAR

Although uncommon, thrombosis of the subclavian vein produces shoulder area pain. It should be considered when engorgement of the veins and swelling are noted in the arm of a patient with shoulder pain. A history of cancer, blood clotting disorders, trauma, or subclavian venous line placement may be present. Also uncommon is aneurysmal dilatation of the subclavian artery, which produces shoulder pain and decreased pulses at the wrist below. These should be worked up by a vascular surgeon.

Avascular necrosis of the humeral head is associated with a history of steroid use, alcoholism, or sickle cell disease. It is properly an intrinsic shoulder problem, yet it is mentioned here because the pain it produces in the early phase of bone infarction is vascular in origin. This is the pain of venous congestion and hypoperfusion of bone. It is deep and severe, toothachelike, and associated with pain on any movement of the glenohumeral joint as well as tenderness of the joint to posterior palpation. Changes early on may not be visible on plain film. Magnetic resonance imaging is the most sensitive test, although a bone scan is nearly always obtained as well to give an idea of the metabolic state of the bone of the humeral head.

---

**REFERENCES**

1. Fishman MC, Hoffman AR, Klausner RD, Rockson SG, Thaler MS. *Medicine.* Philadelphia, Pa: Lippincott; 1981.
2. Hawkins RJ. Cervical spine and shoulder. *Instr Course Lect Am Assoc Orthop Surg.* 1985;34:191–195.

# Chapter 5

# Pharmacologic Treatment of Shoulder Pain

## GENERAL CONSIDERATIONS

The decision to employ drugs, which are chemicals, in the treatment of most chronic shoulder problems, which are mechanical, is made by physicians seeking primarily to relieve symptoms. It is often true that drug therapy is given to relieve pain on a temporary basis while the practitioner tries to correct the problem. Drugs do provide great benefit to many arthritic patients, especially those with underlying metabolic diseases such as inflammatory arthritis and gout. Infectious problems obviously require antibiotics. Posttraumatic and postsurgical pain may be treated effectively with a limited course of narcotic analgesics. The chronic shoulder problems that make up the bulk of most practices do not generally respond so dramatically to the antiinflammatories, however. They do not require antibiotics and, because of their chronicity, should not be treated with narcotics. Injectable steroid preparations may actually cure some conditions, but most often provide only temporary relief of symptoms with the risk of long-term joint and tendon degeneration. Thus, although they are valuable to some, drugs play a limited role in the treatment of the most common chronic shoulder problems.

An understanding of the role of narcotics is important for everyone involved in patient care. Long-term use of narcotics produces tachyphylaxis, or the development of resistance of the pain to the effects of the narcotic.[1] Even a relatively small dose of narcotic, such as that found in the commonly used drugs that combine aspirin or acetaminophen (Tylenol) with codeine or its synthetic analogs, will produce this effect if taken chronically. Tachyphylaxis begins to appear within approximately 10 days of beginning narcotic use, sooner if more drug is being used, later if less. It appears as the failure of the usual dose to produce pain relief. Herein is the important clinical point: It seems exactly as if the underlying problem is getting worse. There is nothing that tells the patient that the pain-producing problem itself is not becoming more intense. The same stimulus produces greater pain the longer a fixed dose of narcotic is used.

Narcotic use after trauma or surgery is routine and generally safe. Narcotic premedication of the surgical patient before physical therapy sessions can make short-term range of motion goals much easier to achieve. Narcotics for chronic or undiagnosed shoulder pain, however, are apt to produce the tachyphylactic effect, which results in net worsening of pain with loss of motivation and therapeutic confidence. If this phenomenon is suspected, tactful communication with the prescribing physician is needed.

## NONSTEROIDAL ANTIINFLAMMATORY AGENTS

The class of nonsteroidal antiinflammatory drugs (NSAIDs) is large and getting larger. There are currently some 40 different NSAIDs available in the United States. Aspirin is one of them, although its side effect profile is quite high in comparison to the other commonly used drugs. Two other nonprescription NSAIDs are ibuprofen and naproxen. These drugs all carry the risk of stomach and duodenal irritation and ulceration in sensitive patients. People who have had ulcers or gastritis generally should not be given them. Misoprostol (Cytotec) is used specifically to protect the patient from the gastrointestinal side effects of the NSAIDs. In the author's practice, misoprostol itself has had a high rate of complications, the most frequent of which has been diarrhea. The kidneys and liver may also be harmed by long-term use of the NSAIDs, especially in older patients and those on certain antihypertensive medications. Despite these problems, it is unusual to find a shoulder patient who has not used NSAIDs at some time because they are available without prescription.

A common misconception among patients is that NSAIDs can mask pain sufficiently to render physical examination signs negative that would otherwise be present, thus confounding the examiner's ability to determine the diagnosis properly. With the exception of some acute inflammatory conditions, such as gout or calcific tendinitis, these drugs do not have nearly enough efficacy to do this. The type of pain for which NSAIDs have the greatest effectiveness is often termed periosteal. These drugs all act by disrupting the production of prostaglandins, short-lived signal molecules that are involved in the local modulation of a host of tissue responses. Osteoarthritic pain, thought to be created by localized mechanical stress and resultant inflammation, is typically of this type, and it often responds nicely to these agents. Glenohumeral and acromioclavicular arthritics should be tried on these if no contraindications are found. Impingement pain may have an inflammatory component as well. It is therefore worthwhile trying these drugs on impingers. The pain associated with shoulder subluxation, loose bodies, nerve root compression, or an established rotator cuff tear is not likely to be helped by long-term NSAID treatment.

Many of the NSAIDs are like aspirin and inhibit the normal clotting of blood by preventing the aggregation of platelets. These are usually withheld before elective surgery to prevent excessive bleeding. There is a role for the NSAIDs in the postoperative patient, however. The NSAIDs are often quite useful in decreasing the swelling and inflammation associated with postsurgical range and strengthening exercise. They are an important adjunct to the antiswelling modalities, especially because the shoulder's deep submuscular location and excellent vascularity render thermal and electrical modalities less efficient.

Scientifically choosing one NSAID from among the many available is difficult for the physician. The choice of agent is based on the individual physician's experience with the drugs and some differences in the way they are metabolized, the dosing schedules, the individual patient's side effect history, cost, and concomitant medications being taken. It is clearly true that some agents work better than others for a given patient, and thus a few different ones should be tried before one gives up on them entirely. There is no generally recognized hierarchy among the NSAIDs as to which are the most effective relievers of pain. The shoulder patient on NSAIDs should therefore be treated as any other; it is only in rare cases that these drugs can supplant the need for physical treatment.

## STEROIDAL AGENTS

The glucocorticoids share a common chemical structure with the naturally produced hormones that are involved in the organism's response to stress. The sex hormones androgen and estrogen share a similar structure and are indeed steroids that are commonly used as drugs. The present discussion is limited to the powerful antiinflammatories of the glucocorticoid class because they are far more likely to be utilized in the specific treatment of shoulder problems.

Systemic steroids, given by mouth or injection, are the most effective means available of decreasing inflammatory response throughout the entire body. The magnitude of this effect is demonstrated by the fact that normally severe abdominal pain associated with infection, such as appendicitis, may be completely absent in a patient on steroids. It is unusual to find an inflammatory condition that does not respond, at least temporarily, to high doses of steroids. The level of side effects associated with their use, however, is so high that it is also unusual to find a patient for whom any other viable means of symptom control exists on long-term steroid therapy.

Discussions of the side effects of long-term steroid therapy fill many volumes of past and current medical literature. Psychosis, hyperglycemia, increased susceptibility to infection, decreased healing ability, anemia, weight gain, osteoporosis, loss of strength, and lethargy are but a few. Pertinent to the physical treatment of the shoulder patient are significantly increased tissue fragility and decreased ability to strengthen muscle, bone, and tendon. The inflammatory response to local injury or stress is, in one sense, physiologic. It starts the reactions that end in healing, scarring, and strengthening in nearly every tissue in which these changes can occur. The danger of interrupting inflammation systemically can be appreciated in light of this fact.

Patients on long-term steroid treatment are likely to have an autoimmune disease such as rheumatoid arthritis or chronic lung disease. The most important concept to be stressed in their treatment is that it must be gentle and slow. Steroid-treated bone is weak. Skin, muscle, and ligament have decreased mechanical strength and can tear if treatment is too vigorous. Sprains and fractures tend to heal slowly, and muscle strengthening takes longer. This notwithstanding, fractures eventually do heal, and the muscles will strengthen with persistence. It is important not to give up on the steroid-dependent patient in therapy.

Parenteral steroid therapy for shoulder pain is generally used to treat acute, inflammatory disease such as gout, calcific tendinitis, or a flare-up of rheumatoid or psoriatic arthritic disease. The most commonly used dosing pattern is called a pulse; starting with a high daily dose for a few days (up to a week), the daily dose is decreased to low levels and then stopped. This is done to avoid the side effects of long-term therapy. During the period on high-dose therapy (the initial few days), the antiinflammatory effect of the drugs is maximal. There is often good pain relief and even euphoria associated with the high daily dose. If there is an element of frozen shoulder (adhesive capsulitis) being treated, this high-dose interval is a good time to push aggressively for increased motion goals because the normal tissue reactions to capsular stretching and lysis of intraarticular and pericapsular adhesions are blunted. Although the steroid is not an anesthetic, the pain of manipulation does seem to be decreased by high-dose steroid therapy. As the dose comes down, the sense of well-being and the antiinflammatory effect do as well. The physician often warns that when the dose is finally stopped there may be a day or two of mental depression. Patients often report that these are bad days in therapy as well, with increased pain, muscle weakness, and stiffness. An awareness of the temporary nature of these reactions can make them more tolerable. Although not routine, the steroid pulse is used frequently, especially by rheumatologists. By knowing its timing and therapeutic implications, the therapist can utilize its effect to maximum advantage.

Parenteral steroid therapy is occasionally administered as one or more intramuscular injections of long-acting steroid compounds. The data regarding blood levels and the physiologic effects of this vary, but in general a short period of low-level effects is attained this way. Hospitalized patients on intravenous steroids will have their shoulder problems affected in the same way as if the steroids were taken orally. Because the steroids are all fat soluble, little difference in effect is observed among the various methods of steroid administration. It is rather the total dose taken over a given time period that determines the clinical effect.

## LOCAL INJECTIONS

Powerful local effects can be obtained by local steroid injections. As is described under the individual disease categories, many conditions around the shoulder may be successfully treated with local injection therapy using steroid preparations. Some general principles must be kept in mind regarding this type of treatment, however.

First, the potential dangers of injection therapy must be appreciated by both physician and patient. Side effects from local injections are definitely rare. Occurrences after injection are often thought to be caused by the injection when there is little reason to believe this. Reactions and side effects do occur, however, and recognizing them early does help minimize their morbidity.

The most common side effect after a steroid injection is the flare reaction. This is simply an increase in pain and stiffness in the injected area.[2] It seems to be more common after injection of the long-lasting steroid preparations, which are suspensions of solid crystals. It also seems somewhat more common in patients who have exhibited neuropathic or myofascial pain or cutaneous hypersensitivity in the past. The flare reaction may be mild and treatable by reassurance and local application of ice for a day, or it may be severe, requiring narcotics and 5 to 7 days to abate. It is thought to be caused by tissue response to the solid crystals themselves or possibly to extravasated blood from the injecting needle. It would seem logical that the local antiinflammatory effect of the steroid itself would quell this type of response, and well it might because the flare eventually subsides on its own.

Ascertaining that the increase in local pain and inflammation is caused by a flare response and not a local infection brought in by the injecting needle is important but difficult. Knowing that good sterile technique was used in giving the injection is one comfort. The physical examination should be closely followed for local signs of infection, the classic three being tumor (increasing swelling at the injection site), dolor (increasing pain and tenderness), and rubor (increasing redness and warmth). Blood tests for infection may be necessary if suspicion is rising. White blood cell counts, sedimentation rate, and C-reactive protein values will tend to be elevated in the presence of local infection. Clinical judgment is still required to make the diagnosis of local infection after injection because all these parameters may be elevated by underlying disease. Infection is rare after intramuscular injection, somewhat less rare after bursal and peritendinous injection, and still less rare after intraarticular injections of steroids. It is overall an uncommon occurrence; many physiatrists and surgeons have given thousands of injections over their careers without reporting a single infection. Increased pain after an injection is thus far more likely to be caused by a flare response. Infection should nonetheless be kept in mind for it is far easier to treat early on.

Local depigmentation of skin after steroid injection therapy is not uncommon and may be objectionable, especially to dark-skinned people. This is more likely to occur if the steroid was deposited close to the skin. Little can be done to correct this, and dark-skinned patients are best warned of the possibility before steroid injection.

The most serious complications associated with injection of long-lasting steroid preparations are related to the steroids' tendency to blunt the normal healing responses in tendon and periarticular tissues. Tendon ruptures after even a single peritendinous injection have been described in many anatomic locations.[3-7] Although it is certainly true that the peritendinous inflammatory process for which the injection was given is itself a common cause of tendon rupture, the possibility exists that a given rupture might not have occurred if the local steroid had not been administered. In shoulder practice a common question is, How many of these steroid injections around the rotator cuff can be given safely? There is no scientific answer at present. For chronic subacromial impingement in the absence of a rotator cuff tear, three injections within a given 12-month period is a maximum generally held by many orthopaedists.

The tendons that make up the rotator cuff do exhibit healing and scarring reactions under the proper conditions. Although it is nearly impossible for a full-thickness tear to heal without surgery, partial-thickness tears (which may be thought of as abrasions of the cuff) definitely do heal when impingement is stopped. It is for this reason that the use of subacromial steroid injections for patients with impingement is neither universal nor trouble free. Sudden, traumatic rupture of the rotator cuff is not rare. It is likely that the cuff has been attenuated by chronic acromial impingement. It is possible that the cuff has been weakened further by multiple steroid injections with failure of repeated microtrauma to heal.

It has been reliably demonstrated that the uptake of nutrient sugars by fibroblasts in culture is decreased by administration of steroids.[8] It is the fibroblast that is responsible for production of collagen fibers and ultimate healing of collagenous tissues, such as rotator cuff tendon. It therefore seems likely that the high local concentrations of steroid produced by local injection inhibit this cell's function and thus inhibit strengthening and healing of partial tears of the cuff. The phenomenon of sudden, traumatic cuff rupture has not, however, been shown to occur with greater frequency in the population that has had many injections.

The effect of multiple steroid injections on articular cartilage is variable[7] and difficult to isolate in clinical practice because all patients receiving these injections have some type of arthritis, itself a disease of articular cartilage, to begin with. Steroid injections into inflamed joints profoundly affect synovial blood flow and hypertrophy. Symptomatic relief of joint pain is common and can be complete. The abundant, inflamed synovium that can be palpated at the posterior joint line of an acutely painful rheumatoid shoulder will often disappear after an intraarticular steroid injection. This hot, acutely painful joint is, however, the type that the orthopaedist worries most about seeding with an infection or accelerating the articular surface destruction with injections of steroid.

There is a typical appearance of the joint that has been injected multiple times. Yellowing of the remaining articular cartilage and weakening or atrophy of the capsule and pericapsular ligamentous structures are familiar to every orthopaedist performing arthroplasty on these joints. Although these are diseased joints to begin with, the steroid injections are not without morbidity. Within the arthritic joint, the use of injectable steroids should be considered a temporizing, symptomatic measure. Osteoarthritics benefit far less than rheumatoids from glenohumeral injections. Acromioclavicular arthritics of all types may get up to 6 months of pain diminution.

The injection of long-acting steroid compounds into muscular nodes or trigger points is a well established and almost completely mysterious therapy.[9] These tender points occur commonly in the trapezius area. They are often associated with impingement and may disappear if this is relieved. When they are not related to the shoulder or cervical spine, they may be effectively treated with local massage, insonation, or electrical modalities. If these are ineffective, direct injection of the tender points with local anesthetics and steroids can be completely effective in eliminating their symptoms. What these points are and what the injections do to render them less painful are completely unclear. A number of fine texts on injection therapy highlight its use around the shoulder.[10,11]

A steroid injection into a bursal space, node, or peritendinous location should generally not be made until it has been determined that an anesthetic injection at the same location produces symptomatic relief or diminution of the characteristic local tenderness at that point. Because so little is understood of the actual mechanism of action of locally injected steroids, the utmost attention must be paid to effects created by the local anesthetic injected at the same point. The fact that an area of local tenderness has been rendered nontender is less likely to predict good response to a steroid injection than the observation of the local anesthetic injection temporarily eliminating the patient's symptoms and provocative signs.

In practice, the majority of steroid injections performed around the shoulder are into the subacromial bursa and acromioclavicular joint. The surety with which diagnoses at these locations can be made on physical examination prompts many physicians to give steroid injections simultaneously with local anesthetic agents for a combined diagnostic injection test and local steroid injection.

## REFERENCES

1. Goodman L, Gillman A, Goodman-Gillman A. *The Pharmacologic Basis of Therapeutics.* New York, NY: Macmillan; 1980; 75, 505–508.

2. Travell J. Factors affecting pain of injection. *JAMA.* 1955;158:368–371.

3. Ford LT, DeBender J. Tendon rupture after local steroid injection. *South J Med.* 1979;72:827–830.

4. Ismail AM, Balakrishnan R, Rajakumar MK. Rupture of the patellar tendon after steroid infiltration. *J Bone Joint Surg Br.* 1969;51:503–505.

5. Lee HB. Avulsion and rupture of the tendon calcaneus after injection of hydrocortisone. *Br J Med.* 1957;2:395.

6. Uitto J, Teir H, Mustakallio KK. Corticosteroid induced inhibition of biosynthesis of human skin collagen. *Biochem Pharmacol.* 1972;21:2161–2167.

7. Salter RB, Gross A, Hall JH. Hydrocortisone arthropathy; an experimental investigation. *Can Med Assoc J.* 1967;97:374–377.

8. Gray ET. Effect of glucocorticoid on hexose uptake by mouse fibroblast. *Biochemistry.* 1971;10:277–284.

9. Travell J, Rinzler S. The myofascial genesis of pain. *Postgrad Med.* 1952;11:425–434.

10. Cyriax J. *Textbook of Orthopedic Medicine.* 5th ed. Baltimore, Md: Williams & Wilkins; 1969; 1.

11. Steinbrocker O, Neustadt DH. *Aspiration and Injection Therapy in Arthritis and Musculoskeletal Disorders.* Hagerstown, Md: Harper and Row; 1972; 39–66.

# Chapter 6

# The Roles of Physical Medicine and Orthopaedics in Treatment of the Shoulder Patient

## CONSERVATIVE TREATMENT

That which constitutes conservative treatment of a given health problem is subjective. It depends on who is treating and, increasingly, on who is being treated. There are few health care professionals who would admit to being against conservative treatment. Traditionally, however, this term has implied no surgery, no medications with many side effects, and no "alternative" therapies such as acupuncture, aroma therapy, chiropractic, or herbal therapy. This has left physical therapy as "conservative treatment" in the minds of many, including some physical therapists and physiatrists as well as many insurance companies.

Many insurance companies today routinely require a patient to have undergone conservative treatment, meaning physical therapy, for 6 weeks before granting authorization for orthopaedic surgery. Underlying this requirement is the assumption by these insurers that a number of patients will be forced to undergo physical therapy and either will improve sufficiently so as not to require the expensive surgery or will not improve and thus lose confidence in the surgeon who prescribed the therapy, leave his or her care, and go to someone else who might not recommend the expensive surgery. There is also an assumption that the treating physician will tend to recommend the expensive surgery even though the problem could be adequately treated with physical therapy alone, for his or her own financial gain.

Barring an unexplained enthusiasm for rehabilitative therapy among health insurance executives, the companies' requirement that physical therapy fail before surgical treatment is initiated is based on the principle that physical therapy can take the place of surgical therapy and is less expensive. The physician who recommends surgery when physical therapy alone is clearly adequate treatment is considered by most wrong and not treating conservatively. This concept is generally well appreciated. It is important to understand the converse situation, however: Nonsurgical procedures are not always the most conservative. Because so many of the common ailments about the shoulder respond well to physical methods, this issue is especially important in the care of the shoulder patient.

Acute, traumatic rupture of the entire rotator cuff may be treated with 6 weeks of range of motion and strengthening therapy with some hope of improvement of strength through recruitment of other muscles. The prognosis for this condition when treated with early surgical repair is quite good. This prognosis becomes worse with every month that the tear is not repaired. Physical therapy here is not the safest treatment for the shoulder, nor should it be considered the most conservative because, compared to surgery, it has a much greater likelihood of resulting in a permanent loss of function. Nonsurgical treatment is recommended only for patients who are not likely to miss active shoulder motion, such as the frail elderly under institutional care.

For the practitioner who is honestly and intelligently working to treat his or her patient, the practice of conservative treatment today may include cessation of physical methods and even the recommendation of surgery. Understanding the pathophysiology of the problem under treatment enables the practitioner to address the underlying issue in this type of situation. Most simply, it is the question of conservative versus optimal treatment. *Staphylococcus aureus*, inflecting the glenohumeral joint cavity, is optimally treated by surgical drainage, hospitalization, and intravenous antibiotics. More conservative treatment might be repeated needle aspiration and oral antibiotics as an outpatient. Most conservative would possibly be rest, herbal teas with antibiotic claims, and application of hot packs. The latter two plans would clearly be dangerous to follow because of the strong possibility of joint destruction and even death that they would create. These two more conservative plans would probably produce some symptomatic relief at first. They could meet with the approval of a large number of nonsurgical health care practitioners and would be far less likely to be challenged by insurance companies' preauthorization agents than the first plan's prolonged hospitalization with a number of expensive surgical procedures. Most approving might be the patient himself or herself, a health-conscious individual with a healthy suspicion of physicians who finds the concept of being cut open and kept in a hospital bed on dangerous drugs ridiculous, together with the mumbo-jumbo about having gotten some germ from going to the dentist. Amidst these factors, the honest and intelligent practitioner must insist that only the optimal course of therapy be followed. A practitioner in physical medicine who knows the signs and symptoms of a septic shoulder must raise the alarm and recommend against conservative treatment in this case. It is not the role of this practitioner simply to render conservative treatment. Optimal treatment ought to be the goal of every member of the health care team.

There are obviously many instances in which the risks of conservative treatment are not so clear as they are in the cases of septic arthritis and complete cuff avulsion. Because shoulder patients are often underdiagnosed and misdiagnosed by physicians who prescribe evaluation and treatment in their hospital's physical therapy department, the burden of diagnosis and treatment recommendations for shoulder patients falls more heavily on the practitioners in physical medicine. The practitioner should therefore understand all treatments that are available for the shoulder patient, not just the conservative ones that he or she is responsible for rendering.

## DEFINING TREATMENT GOALS

High-quality care is delivered when all members of the health care team have the same goals on both short- and long-term bases. Patient, therapist, physiatrist, medical doctor, and surgeon, working toward the same goal, have a much greater chance of realizing that goal than an individual faction within this group working alone. Shoulder problems are often complex enough to make reference to this kind of health care platitude worthwhile. It is common in shoulder practice for fragmentation and concentration on different goals to compromise clinical results.

An example is often seen in the course of a surgically treated patient with a two- or three-part proximal humerus fracture. The surgeon, following radiographs and highly concerned about the stability of the fracture construct, is at odds with the therapist, who is concerned with achieving motion and strength goals, and both are at odds with the patient, who is most concerned about how much all this is costing and whether the miserable pain will ever stop. The result of this might be that the surgeon, not trusting the therapist to perform true passive motion, holds off rehabilitation for an extra month to let fracture healing improve the stability of the surgical construct. This results in extra stiffness, which the therapist attacks too aggressively, producing an intolerable level of pain. The patient, seeking to avoid this pain and save the money he or she is paying the therapist, then skips many therapy sessions and ends up with a stiff, painful, and weak shoulder. This poor result might have been avoided had each of the three team members been aware of the goals, concerns, and abilities of the others.

Most shoulder patients are treated to achieve a combination of pain relief and functional improvement. The goals of individuals may be extraordinarily disparate despite their having the same diagnosis. The first job of the health care provider is to focus on what these goals are. An older patient with diabetes may need restoration of motion to a frozen shoulder sufficient only to permit axillary and perineal hygiene. The short- and long-term goals need not include any strengthening or endurance. This patient's 20-year-old grandchild could present with the same diagnosis (frozen shoulder) and yet actually require that his or her extension range in abduction be increased to supraphysiologic values and make use of sport-specific training with isokinetic apparatus to achieve the functional goal of throwing a different baseball pitch.

It is a good practice for shoulder surgeons to specify exact motion and strength goals with each therapy prescription. A common terminology promotes efficient communication among the various members of the team. "PROM prog to 120/45/L1, AA cuff str adv to concentric ant cuff iso v gravity" is a typical prescription. Translated, this means passive range of motion, progressive increase to 120° forward elevation, 45° external rotation, internal rotation to the first lumbar segment, active assisted rotator cuff strengthening with advancement to concentric anterior cuff (supraspinatus) isolation to the point that the arm can be raised against gravity (Figure 6–1).

Patient motivation is improved by setting and reaching attainable short-term goals. Therapists who are not given them by a prescribing physician should set them themselves. For easily quantifiable parameters such as motion and strength, it is a relatively straightforward thing to pick goals that seem to be attainable in a given session, week, or month. Shoulder patients may have functional or prophylactic objectives that are more difficult around which to tailor therapeutic parameters.

Just as some algebraic functions approach their limits asymptomatically, never quite reaching a set level, patients in therapy for prophylactic reasons (to prevent future shoulder dislocations, for instance) may never reach the level of 100% confidence that another similar event (dislocation in this example) will not occur. Treatment goals for this type of patient may not be definable in terms of motion or strength. Neither does the concept of stopping exercise after reaching an arbitrary goal seem appropriate. Still, it is not practical to continue in outpatient physical therapy for the rest of one's life, so a decision must be made. The faculty, generally called clinical judgment, employed to make this type of decision well is in large part sensitivity to patients' verbal and physical feedback to questioning, training goals, and physical examination.

The dislocator (to follow the example given), when properly rehabilitated, has a week when the shoulder starts to feel less sloppy. Internal rotation

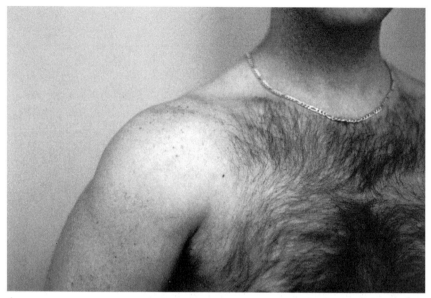

A

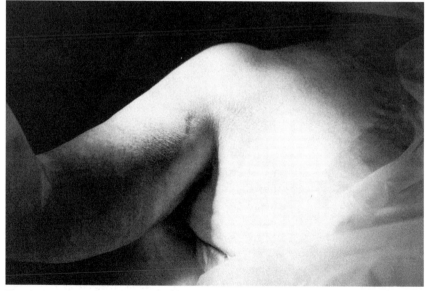

B

**Figure 6–1 (A)** Strong athletic shoulder patient, a weightlifter after surgical repair of a complete cuff avulsion. A diagnostic and therapeutic contrast with the **(B)** weak and debilitated shoulder patient.

strength may not change at all that week. Ranges may stay exactly the same. It is likely that some type of proprioception may be reestablished, but this has not been proved. That week the careful therapist may notice that the scapulothoracic rhythm looks more like the other side's. The sense of wellness in the shoulder may be hard to describe, but to the practitioner who has been working hard with a well-motivated patient it is usually quite obvious. This is a signpost of the asymptotic goal toward which the entire health care team works. It is likely to be noticed first by the shoulder patient's therapist.

Relief of pain, restoration of full motion and strength, and the vague sense of joint stability or normalized joint position sense may all be thought of by practitioners as ultimate goals of treatment. The underlying goal of patients themselves is usually simpler, however: They want to be able to forget about their shoulder. A normal joint, muscle, or organ is unlikely to be the subject of much consideration by its owner. It may be difficult with some patients to undo the great concentration on the shoulder that the course of treatment has created. More so than with other joints, "shoulder consciousness," once created, can be long lived. The pitfall to be avoided is letting heightened shoulder consciousness drive treatment. Just as it is wrong to treat for reasons that are purely financial or emotional, it is wrong to let a patient's zeal for perfection drive one to treat a normal joint. Although sensitivity to patient complaints is of the utmost importance, it ought not to be to the patient's own detriment. After a long and successful treatment course, quite a strong bond can form between the patient and those treating him or her. It is the final goal of successful treatment to recognize that it has been successful and thus is no longer needed.

## INDICATIONS FOR PHYSICAL THERAPY

Much more so than most therapists, the surgeon is used to specifying indications for treatment, meaning those factors that both prompt and justify the course of treatment he or she chooses. It is good practice for all members of the health care team to maintain awareness of the specific indications for which they are rendering their treatment. "I've gotten this prescription that says to do it" is generally insufficient as an indication for the holder of a professional license. Working under the direction of a physician, a therapist may rely on information that he or she did not request, such as radiographs, because primary responsibility for diagnosis rests with a physician. The most basic set of indications for physical therapy must therefore include a diagnosis. Responsibility for physical examination does rest with therapists, however, and a physical examination that is inconsistent with the diagnosis is cause for communication with the referring physician.

Not all shoulder patients require physical treatment, but the majority do at some point in their treatments. Indications for physical treatment in general are therefore quite broad. The indications for the specific treatment being rendered should be kept in mind at all times. This is especially true regarding the use of modalities. Patients are often sent for ultrasound and continue to show up for treatment for weeks after the specific indication for that treatment, which may have been a painful trapezius spasm, is no longer present. There is then a good chance that the patient and therapist are wasting their time with ultrasound. If the reason for the trapezius spasm was subacromial cervicalgia, those therapy sessions would have been better spent working on strengthening of the humeral head depressors, an appropriate treatment for which the indications were still present. The most effective practitioners in physical medicine stay constantly aware of the specific indications for the treatments they are giving.

## INDICATIONS FOR SURGERY

In practice, an orthopaedic surgeon's development of the set of indications for each of the various operations that he or she performs is a complex and personal process. The individual surgeon's experience, diagnostic judgment, and technical ability influence his or her indications strongly. Pertinent here is the importance of failure of conservative means of treatment as an indication for surgery.

The vast majority of elective shoulder surgeries (done by ethical surgeons) are indicated only after physical treatment fails to control the patient's symptoms. This is easily understood. Less straightforward is the common problem with shoulder patients of reliance on therapy to prevent recurrence of symptoms. In these situations, a decision is ultimately faced: to go on with therapy, albeit intermittently, for the rest of the patient's life, or to correct the problem surgically and, one hopes, stop the therapy. This situation often occurs in the treatment of subacromial impingement, in which supraphysiologic levels of cuff tone can hold down the impingement phenomenon and its pain but as soon as exercise is stopped the tone disappears and the pain returns.

To be avoided in these situations is the adversarial stance that the situation may create between the surgeon and the physical therapist. Surgeon or therapist may start this by encouraging the patient to work hard at therapy, threatening an operation if he or she does not. Presentation of surgery as a punishment for poor therapy compliance is usually unwise. The reasons for this are readily apparent. The decision to have surgery or continue with treatments is ultimately the patient's. The responsibility for obtaining a good result belongs to the practitioners (surgeon and therapist), however, and their ability to do so may be compromised by communication to the patient that the therapist has failed in his or her attempt to "protect" the patient from the surgeon. It should always be stressed to the patient that he or she will have an even greater need for physical therapy after surgery and that the goals of both surgeon and therapist treating the shoulder are exactly the same.

## PREHABILITATION, REHABILITATION, MAINTENANCE, AND TRAINING

These concepts need to be clear to physician and therapist because they involve short- and long-term goals, indications, and expectations.

### Prehabilitation

This term usually implies strengthening and stretching in anticipation of an insult, usually surgery. A prehabilitative function is served by most rotator cuff and shoulder girdle strengthening for a number of reasons. First, surgery is often technically superior in the patient who has done long-term shoulder exercises for these structures. The mechanical strength of the remaining rotator cuff tissues, deltoid muscle, and capsular structures of the glenohumeral joint does seem to be superior in patients who have worked hard preoperatively. This means that they are easier to delineate and manipulate, hold sutures more securely, and probably heal a bit faster. Surgeons worry less about soft tissue failures, such as the deltoid muscle pulling off the acromion or the repaired rotator cuff or subscapularis pulling off the humerus, in an athletic shoulder that has done effective preoperative exercise. Second, because the tissues are stronger to begin with, it is generally possible to advance strengthening and motion goals more quickly after surgery in the well-prehabilitated shoulder. Third, because most of the postsurgical exercises are fairly similar to the presurgical ones, the patient is more adept at them in the postoperative period, when he or she is dealing with added pain and weakness.

When a new shoulder patient does not seem to be responding to physical treatment and thus begins the consideration of surgery, it is good practice to stress the prehabilitative value of the therapy he or she is doing, both as a motivational device and to have the patient understand the team approach that is used. The "therapy versus surgery" battle lines will not be drawn if this team approach is emphasized. The physical treatments will also not be considered wasted if an operative plan is eventually adopted.

### Rehabilitation

The term implies recovering from the effects of an insult, which, again, may be surgery. Practitioners in physical medicine are well aware of their role in rehabilitative therapy; those in orthopaedics and internal medicine may not be as understanding. In contrast to the prehabilitative situation, it is the physicians who need to be "kept on the team" in the rehabilitative setting. Implicit in the rehabilitation concept is a definite improvement that is expected over the course of treatment. In treating postsurgical shoulder patients, more often than not there is an unwelcome period of functional deterioration that may be accompanied by increased pain. The physical medicine practitioner who conveys a sense of trust in the surgeon and the surgical procedure performed does much to help the patient through these periods. The surgeon needs to play an active role during these periods of temporary dehabilitation, sometimes by changing or decreasing physical therapy, changing medication, or utilizing bracing.

These setback periods are so common as to be the norm for patients in postoperative rehabilitation. They are not to be considered surgical complications. Surgical repairs can and do sometimes fail, and early and late surgical complications may ruin what seemed to be a good result. Although the physical medicine practitioner must be able to recognize these occurrences, it is properly the surgeon's role to diagnose and treat surgical failures and complications. It is by no means appropriate for physical medicine practitioners to trivialize or hide surgical complications, but it is devastating for the patient to be told that a surgical complication has occurred when in fact it has not. Trust in the entire team is lost, and the psychic effect is for the patient to anticipate greater and greater symptoms without hope of cure. It is also unlikely that a physical medicine practitioner will have seen enough surgical complications to be able to diagnose them reliably. There is a good chance that what he or she feels is a retearing of the repaired cuff is early overuse or eccentric stretch or that the wound infection is a sterile inflammatory reaction to absorbable suture material. Regardless of whether there truly has been a complication, the job of announcing it to the patient and then dealing with it belongs to the surgeon. Much anguish may be avoided by observing this rule.

The person with whom concerns about surgical complications and failures should be discussed first is always the surgeon. The surgeon should then evaluate and make treatment recommendations accordingly, explaining the situation to the patient. A therapist who announces that a surgical failure or complication has occurred can seriously compromise the patient's rehabilitation potential, independent of the presumed complication itself.

### Maintenance

The idea of maintenance therapy, designed to prevent relapse or deterioration, has greater appeal to many patients who have just successfully completed a course of physical treatment for a painful shoulder problem. It does